Standing on an Apple Box

Standing on an Apple Box

The Story of a Girl among the Stars

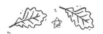

AISHWARYAA R. DHANUSH

FOREWORD BY
SHWETA BACHCHAN NANDA

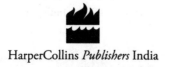

HarperCollins *Publishers* India

First published in hardback in India in 2016 by
HarperCollins *Publishers* India

Copyright © Aishwaryaa R. Dhanush 2016

P-ISBN: 978-93-5264-175-8
E-ISBN: 978-93-5264-176-5

2 4 6 8 10 9 7 5 3 1

HarperCollins *Publishers*

A-75, Sector 57, Noida, Uttar Pradesh 201301, India
1 London Bridge Street, London, SE1 9GF, United Kingdom
Hazelton Lanes, 55 Avenue Road, Suite 2900, Toronto, Ontario M5R 3L2
and 1995 Markham Road, Scarborough, Ontario M1B 5M8, Canada
25 Ryde Road, Pymble, Sydney, NSW 2073, Australia
195 Broadway, New York, NY 10007, USA

Typeset in 11/14 Adobe Jenson Pro at
SÜRYA, New Delhi

Printed and bound at
Thomson Press (India) Ltd

This book is dedicated to all those celebrity children who manage to retain their sanity and sensibility through it all.

Contents

Foreword

I first met Aishwaryaa a year ago, when she accompanied her father to a football match, and I had gone with mine. We took our seats behind them as they cheered and clapped their teams on, like excited boys. I could almost read her thoughts. She was thrilled that her father had got an opportunity to let his hair down for a while in the company of a friend and, at least for a couple of hours, the world's eyes were not trained on him. I know this because I was thinking the very same thing about my father.

When she called to ask if I would write the foreword to her first book, Aishwaryaa mentioned feeling an affinity to me, as one might with someone who has shared similar life experiences. A few hours later, she very efficiently sent me a rough draft of her book. That evening, as I sat reading, I caught myself smiling at some parts, nodding my head in agreement at others. It was all so relatable. These could have been vignettes from my own life, experiences I had shared with my own father. It's uncanny how similar our trajectories are. Our fathers have been colleagues and friends for years, our families have always had the highest regard for each other. It's easy to see why we have so much in common, not just in our public lives but in our private moments as well.

What the book beautifully brings to life is the story of a regular girl growing up in a not-so-regular home. The story of a mother bringing up her daughters in the gargantuan shadow of their father and being able to bring them up as unspoiled by it as possible. Very often we watch our idols on screen and they take on the superhuman qualities of the characters they portray. What *Standing on an Apple Box* does is lift the curtain and give you a peek at the men and women behind the makeup and the family units that helped to make them what they are. The stories from Aishwaryaa's childhood are charming in their simplicity and I couldn't get enough of the escapades from the life of one of the world's most recognized men. Though her father is an extraordinary man in every sense of the word, it is the ordinary rituals that he practises in his life, whether for himself or his family, that very clearly are the secrets to his success, as his daughter tells it. Her account of him manages to make a revered icon accessible and, in doing so, she gives hordes of fans the most authentic version of their hero.

This book is the story of a father and daughter, an icon and his fans, a man and his family. What I like best about it is that it is real, from the heart, and bone honest.

SHWETA BACHCHAN NANDA

Standing on an Apple Box

Movie sets have been a part of my life since I can remember. It is a universe unto itself. Reality does not lose its hold, but becomes twisted. The pace is different, sometimes day is turned into night, summer to rain and your humble, quiet father turns into a rowdy-bashing, dialogue-delivering superstar.

Once, a girl joined the film industry intent on becoming a cinematographer. (Yes, times have changed; all women do not want to become actresses.) She was talented and hard-working and was soon hired to assist a renowned Director of Photography (DP in movie lingo). On the first day of the shoot, excited and nervous, she approaches her boss, who is busy setting up things.

'Cut that backlight a little more. Hey, you! Get the skimmer on this one. You there! Fix a 2 kv here …' He glances at her and says softly, 'You. Baby.'

She looks around and cannot spot a baby, nor does she recall the script having any baby. Running to one of the many assistant directors, she asks, 'Is there a baby in this scene? He is asking for the baby!' The AD, who is enjoying a quiet smoke before the madness began, panics. 'There is no baby in today's scene! Oh my god! Is there? Where will we get a baby now!'

He whips out his phone and the girl decides she has to clarify the matter and walks back, but before she can ask anything, the cameraman points to her. 'Baby... go... now!'

She backs away. Is she being dismissed? Did he just call her baby! It's her first day at work and her boss has just called her baby and asked her to leave. Confusion prevails. Is he being chauvinistic, sleazy, dismissive? She wants to burst into tears but that would just reinforce the usual misogyny.

Now you must be thinking this girl was being an utter idiot. But remember the aura surrounding movies, remember this is a young girl with stars in her eyes, coming to work for the first time in an industry not exactly known for welcoming women behind the scenes with open arms. It can scramble even a professional's brains. But by now she is at least sure there is no actual baby involved in the scene.

The cameraman is getting impatient. He gestures to a more experienced assistant and says, 'Baby, da...'

Wow! Tears forgotten, the girl tries to wrap her head around this new scenario. He called the guy baby too.

The assistant calmly goes over to a bunch of equipment and brings out a large light on a stand and props it near the cameraman, who barks, 'Finally!' before getting back to work.

So a movie set even has a language of its own, from the self-explanatory 'crane' to the 'akela', the 'dolly', the 'jimmy jib' and the 'apple box'.

Movies are related to glamour, glitz and everything starry, but movie-making is a hectic, draining, unglamorous business. Anybody who has ever been to a movie set knows this. The magic unfolds slowly, painstakingly, and in small bursts of creativity sandwiched between mind-numbing preparations. To start with, I had very little idea about the glamorous side of the business, but I was always thrilled when visiting a set. And I soon discovered that one of the humblest, yet most versatile pieces of equipment used was not the camera, nor the lights, but a small wooden crate-like box called the 'apple box'. These boxes come in various sizes and are called apple, half apple, quarter apple and pancake, don't ask me why. I have asked a number of people and come up with nothing. One theory is that they were initially sourced from apple orchards where they were used to store apples. The biggest of them are about 20'x12'x8' in size. They are used to store objects to transport to the set, and can be stacked inside each other. So versatile, yet so simple in design!

Apple boxes are also used to increase the height of the camera stand, to support heavy equipment, to make short actors look tall (many a petite female actor has used it [off frame] to match her fellow actor's height, and a few male actors too!). They are used to sit on between shots, to serve tea and coffee, to place equipment, to level equipment, as steps, as ladders, and even as tables to work on. Come to any movie shoot and the light man can be heard shouting for it and some assistant director will be scampering around with it.

When not in use, the other equipment would often turn into playthings for me. The round trolley became a merry-go-round, the crane became a giant wheel. The small crane became a see-saw and I would swing to and fro on the straight trolley. But it was the apple box that accompanied me everywhere.

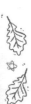

The production assistant would place some snacks for me on it. When I watched Appa on the monitor, I would be sitting on an apple box.

And when one of the most magical moments in my life occurred—I looked through the camera eye and realized instantly and for the first time why movies are magic—I was standing on an apple box.

Today, when I am at a shooting spot and things are going crazy, as they always do, I take a deep breath, drag an apple box to a corner and sit for a moment. Maybe because I was born into and married into the movie business, an apple box is my idea of comfort. Actors, equipment, methods and genres may come and go, but the apple box stays. I know that as long as there are movies there will be madness, but a simple foot-wide, wooden box is all it takes to give me the courage to find a method in it, to find the magic in it, and hopefully find the courage to create a little of that magic—standing on an apple box.

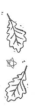

Celebrity Child

One of the most common questions addressed to me is: What is it like being a celebrity child? Even now, when I am anything but a child.

How different is your life? Do you miss having a normal life? Do you feel lucky/unlucky? Don't you think that everything comes easily to you?

And variations of the same.

When I was young, these questions irritated me. I have had this one life and from my point of view, it's normal. Later, I understood the curiosity as the nature of my father's stardom came home to me. The truth was that my father left his stardom and his work at the door when he came into the house. He was our Appa at home, strict when necessary and loving all through. But I learned to answer the questions patiently.

So, what was it like being a celebrity child?

I had a pretty normal childhood, so didn't even realize I was a 'celebrity child'. As I grew up, I felt blessed most of the time. I know there were a lot of responsibilities attached to the tag and I tried my best to understand and act accordingly. (Very diplomatic and correct, I should point out.)

How does it feel to have a superstar as a father?

My father never ever behaves like a superstar at home. For

that matter, he doesn't behave like one anywhere, except in his movies. So it's like having a normal, loving father who is extra busy but otherwise treats us like his little girls.

How different is your life?

It really isn't very different at all. The same twenty-four hours during which we eat, sleep, watch lots of movies, argue, laugh, cry, party, sleep and, of course, work and worry, just the same as everybody else. The only difference being that when we do it, people notice. Particularly in the last decade or so.

Do you have it easy?

Not at all. Everything I do is filtered through the lens of my father's immense talent and success (and now, of course, my husband's). If any doors open, they may have hidden agendas concealed behind them. And believe me when I tell you that unless you have talent, you cannot succeed, no matter who your family is. The first step may be paved, but the rest of the way to any achievement rests solely on your shoulders, and these shoulders carry the extra burden of being compared to two extremely accomplished individuals I am related to by blood and by marriage. The one who gave life to me, and the one I share my life with.

Did you miss out on a normal childhood?

Fortunately not. Most of the credit goes to Amma for having brought us up without any visible signs of my father's stardom. And to Appa, of course, for being the humble person he is, never hinting at his stardom. We never travelled in, or owned, fancy cars (Appa still doesn't). No fancy bags or clothes. We shopped like everyone else in the local showrooms of Madras (now Chennai) and Bangalore. Like any middle-class child of my age, I was unaware of the concept of pocket money and never had any, except the little amounts we were given on festivals and other special occasions. We did frequent restaurants a lot, but were never bothered by anyone. Nobody recognized us (thanks to my father's policy of never releasing any photographs of the family), so we went on the usual temple and beach trips pretty often. We played at Marina beach almost every second day and visited the temples at Adayar and Santhome every week. Food would be packed and brought from home and we would sit in the temple halls, eating and watching people walk by (a common Madras pastime). Amma would sometimes let us eat out and we would walk into the small eateries around the temples and beaches and stuff our faces. There was no Internet and no cell phones for people to click snaps with or take videos, else photos of my gluttony would have kept the world wide web entertained for a long time. Nobody stared, or cared, and we went about our business of growing up, just like all our friends did. Even during any functions that involved Appa, we would sit a few rows behind with trusted uncles, aunts and cousins. Amma did this so that we did not appear in the flurry of photographs inevitably taken of Appa and everyone around him. Most of the other stars sent their children abroad to study and stay out of the public eye. My parents did not want to let us go, so other safeguards were put in place to ensure we had a normal childhood.

I went for summer vacations to Bangalore and stayed at my maternal grandparents' place. We did have lovely birthday parties, but nothing extravagant. We went for movies, ate chaat at Gangotree, binged on junk food at every outing, played checkers late into the night, and that was the extent of the indulgences that came our way.

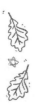

One incident does come to mind that shows how clueless we were. (And how patient Appa often is.)

Polio was a cause that my father supported and he had done

a public service announcement for the same. It was all over television and radio. Many people tried to find some hidden meaning in his support, and coupled with the fact that we were kept away from the public eye, decided that my sister or I had some 'physical issues', maybe even polio.

During this time, one of my father's friends visited with a few friends of his. They were Appa's admirers. One of them, a lady, seemed super excited. Tea and snacks were served and photos taken. We were at home and were called in to say hello to the guests. Most of you would have gone through this: Paraded in front of guests and made to show off what you had learned in school or dance class. Once the 'hello uncle, hello aunty...' were over, the lady asked us to sing a song for them. It wasn't out of the ordinary, so we went ahead and sang some default song that we had been taught at school. Usually after this the adults would get back to their tea and gossip while we filed away to our rooms. But this time the lady applauded and urged us on to sing some more and then she said, 'Now why don't you dance like your father?' Like any kids of that age, we were not immune to being the centre of attention, so we clumsily tried to copy some dance steps we had seen in the movies, completely out of sync but enjoying ourselves. The lady clapped and smiled sweetly, even got up to look closer at us. All the other adults were smiling and we thought we were doing something extraordinary.

It was only later that Appa remarked on what she was really doing. This very pleasant lady had heard the rumours and was checking if they were true. Trying to find out if we had problems talking, walking, etc. Every time we did something, she couldn't hide her surprise and her extreme curiosity pushed her into asking us to do something different. This went on for about half an hour. As kids we were pretty oblivious and thought she was genuinely enjoying our performance. What she really wanted to find out was why Rajinikanth kept his kids hidden away.

As a mother I perfectly understand Appa's reasons for keeping us out of the limelight. And if that lady is anything to go by, he protected us from a lot of heartache. We were able to indulge in the small pleasures that make childhood special, without worrying about the outside world. The situation is diametrically different today. Some of the gossip is so wild, the technology so fast and seamless, I am sure that the polio rumour would have ended in photoshopped images, wild theories and emotional scarring for us. I imagine (I am going to extremes but bear with me, things like this happen) it would have forced my father to release some family photos, and our anonymity, together with our freedom and childhood innocence, would have taken a beating. I am thankful he did not do that or, rather, that his hand was not forced.

Celebrity kids are under so much pressure, it is more surprising when they turn out well than when they don't. I must say I am very impressed with the younger lot that came after me. My kids have the double burden of having famous parents and grandparents. I try my best to shield them at this young age, but I must admit it is difficult. What most people don't understand in their urge to find out more is that celebrity kids are kids too. Too much attention, too much exposure and too much magnifying of their actions can spell disaster. An entire industry revolves around this, and we can see the horrible effects on many famous adults who were exposed to the media incessantly since their childhood, especially in the West.

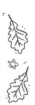

It's wishful thinking on my part, but I wish society would leave these kids alone and not stunt their childhood. Living in Chennai (which is particular about privacy and manners) helps and being vigilant to the point of paranoia, I have even taught my boys to turn their faces away when a stranger photographs them. And I rue the fact that it's not so easy for them to step out for a simple walk to the end of the road for an ice cream or experience the unadulterated joy of running amok in the sands and among the colourful stalls of Marina beach. It's a pleasure that should not be denied to any child living in this city.

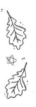

My Father, the Superstar

We love the idea of educating our children. We go to great lengths to ensure they get into the best schools. From registering at birth, queuing up at midnight to get applications, to calling up your third cousin's wife's brother's colleague's grandfather for a recommendation. Then we enrol them in every extracurricular activity or class in the vicinity. I am guilty of this too, though I feel I am doing it for the right reason: to give my children an opportunity to learn a variety of skills. And while running them from one thing to another, I keep in mind a valuable lesson I learned from my father.

I was about five years old and playing by myself in the living room, where Appa sat immersed in some papers. There was a pedestal fan in one corner. Those of you with children know what happens when a toddler and a whirring set of blades meet. My fingers were in dangerous proximity to the fan blades when my father swooped in, much like the heroes he plays on screen, and whipped me away. And like most parents who have had a fright due to their child's inattentiveness, proceeded to give me a scolding. I was not used to seeing an angry Appa, and ran away to cry and sulk in another room.

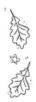

A couple of hours later, as Appa was leaving for a shoot, I, with a normal five-year-old's resilience, came running out to give him a tight hug and a big smile. I don't remember any of this, but in later years Appa recalled the overwhelming sense of guilt and love he felt at that moment. He was struck by the innocence of a child who can forget a frightful scolding and love unconditionally. Most of us would not have recognized this life lesson, but Appa with his innate sense of empathy and humility made this simple episode a learning experience. Many of us would have given the child another lecture on staying out of trouble and spoilt the moment; I know I would have been tempted to. But not Appa. There is, I have always felt, a deep vein of innocence in Appa that helps him to recognize it in others.

It did not stop there; one day Appa came to me and asked permission to use the scene in a movie that had scope for it in the storyline. Remember, this is a traditional Indian father, a movie actor and a very successful personality asking permission from his daughter, long before personal privacy, children's individuality, etc., became buzzwords. Of course my reaction was a resounding Yes!

I didn't even have to think about it, because my Appa had.

The scene with some modifications made it into a movie called *Annamalai*. I like to think that it's the super father in him that translated on to the screen and made him such a beloved superstar.

Sacred Ashes

Appa's spiritual temperament is well known. While most of it is directed inward, there is one thing that embodies his spirituality in his appearance. After his bath in the morning, he smears three lines of vibhuti on his forehead before leaving for work, and this is repeated after his evening bath too, irrespective of whether he is spending the night at home or going out. I don't know if it was my wild childhood imagination or just the result of seeing my father fresh and ready to take on the day or night, mixed with the heavenly fragrance and the gravitas of an ancient ritual, but I thought his face radiated a sense of otherworldly calm every time he placed those three lines on his forehead. I would ape him blindly, placing a small line on my own forehead every morning and night. But I didn't feel any different. So one day, I asked him why it was such an important part of his routine. I expected the answer to be something like, his elder brother had done it before him and he was just following his example—or something similar. But as always, the story turned out to be much more interesting.

Appa had his primary education at Gavipuram Government School. Today, Gavipuram is a bustling Bengaluru suburb, but back then it was a small temple town with the spectacular Gavi Gangadeeswara temple as its focal point. Appa would get up in

13

the morning, have a bath and rush to join his friend Thimmappa, to begin their walk to school. The families expected the boys to take care of each other on their way to and from school. The boys enjoyed each other's company and Appa often helped Thimmappa with his homework.

On their way back, they passed the Gavi Gangadeeswara temple while the first evening puja was in progress, and they would have the prasad before returning home. On weekends too, they would rush to the temple in the evening, just in time for the prasad, and eat it sitting outside. The architecture of that Shiva temple is an instance of ancient Indian engineering at its best. It is carved out of a single granite cave and mysterious stones, whose purpose is lost in time, adorn the entrance. Four monoliths loom above the temple while four pillars, with the sun, the moon, and two Nandis guard the cave. During Makar Shankranthi or the winter solstice, and during the summer solstice, the sun's rays pass precisely between the horns of the Nandis and illuminate the Shiva Linga within the sanctum. As the name suggests, the Gangadeeswara temple is said to have strong ties with Rishikesh and wild theories of tunnels leading all the way north to the holy city from the hill behind the temple are told. I remember when I visited it in my early twenties, there was a stone arch with the Kannada words 'Bagadho Bagilu' (Gateway to Wealth) at the foot of the hill.

To the two primary school boys, the hill was almost a mountain and sitting outside the temple, eating the prasad, the mysterious stones and strange tales were always at the back of their mind. Appa was very curious, but of course no one in the family would allow a ten-year-old to climb the steep, thickly foliated rock face. And so a whole year went by with Appa's curiosity growing day by day. Apart from the elders' warnings, Thimmappa would also not let Appa do anything foolhardy. So he would stare at the hill every morning and evening as he passed, wondering what was at the peak. Another village? Another marvellous temple?

One evening, as Appa was returning from school, he spotted something saffron amidst the green foliage. He ran up to the foot of the hill to get a better look. Two large saffron-coloured sheets were fluttering in the wind, tethered to a line. Appa was excited. There was someone on the hill and he wanted to investigate immediately, but as always Thimmappa dissuaded him and it was getting dark too. He spent the night in agony, thinking about what he had seen. The next day he ran to the foot of the hill on his way to school, but there was nothing to be seen. Tears of disappointment led to an impulsive decision and he started climbing the hill, ignoring Thimmappa's pleas to stop. The slope was slippery and the climb was tough, and he had barely gone a few paces up when one of their schoolmasters spotted the boys. As was the custom in those days, they were given a good spanking and sent to class with a warning to never try climbing the hill again.

Appa couldn't concentrate in class. An entire year of curiosity, followed by the appearance of those mysterious saffron sheets, lit up his now eleven-year-old imagination and sense of adventure. Who had hung them there? What were they doing up there? Were they still up there or had they gone? After school, when he glanced up, there was no flutter of saffron on the hill. His curiosity had also dampened due to Thimmappa's reluctance, the spanking and the elders' warnings and he walked back home feeling miserable.

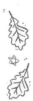

The next morning, as he was getting ready to leave for school, Thimmappa's mother came over to say that he was ill and wouldn't be accompanying him to school that day. My elder uncle decided that Appa was now old enough to walk to school alone, at least this one time, and so Appa set out, still miserable and missing Thimmappa's companionship. The sky was overcast and there was a strong wind blowing. As he reached the gates of the school, big fat drops of rain started falling. Everybody ran to the classrooms, but Appa couldn't help it. He looked up at the hill. There was one saffron cloth, slowly getting drenched in the rain. The first bell had rung, and everyone else had disappeared inside. Without thinking twice, he tossed his schoolbag aside and ran up the slippery slope, the climb made even more precarious because of the rain. The footholds were sharp but something kept him moving. It wasn't an easy climb for an eleven-year-old and it was sheer grit that made him reach the top.

Five trees stood at the summit. Under one of the trees, the ground had been cleared and swept. An old man sat in the clearing and on either side of him stood two young men. All three wore only a saffron cloth wrapped around the waist. To Appa, it appeared as though they were waiting for him. The old man's face radiated serenity and their bodies seemed to be shining through the rain.

Appa narrated the story to us as if it had all happened a few hours earlier, not decades ago. He stood there, as if trying to absorb the energy coming from those three figures. The old man beckoned him forward and he went up to them without hesitation. In his words, it was like an iron nail being pulled by a magnet. The old man smiled and said, 'I was waiting for you, you took some time to reach here.' There was nothing he could say in response, it felt so surreal. The old man reached into a terracotta cup next to him and took out some vibhuti. He then proceeded to smear it all over the little boy's forehead. Appa says he felt something pass through him. A strange sort of vibration, even though the earth and the sky were still. The man gestured for him to leave and without looking back, Appa walked down the hill. His bag lay where he had dropped it. He picked it up and headed to the temple where he sat the entire day. He still doesn't remember how he reached the foot of the hill in that rain. As evening approached, he heard his classmates walk past the temple and decided to head home himself. Nobody had noticed him climb up or come down. The only difference was a forehead smeared with ash.

From the next day onwards, on his way to school, Appa would stop at the temple and ask the priest for some vibhuti and apply it on his forehead. He never saw those saffron-clad men again.

I listened to Appa's story with a sense of awe. At eleven, someone had awakened the latent spiritualism in my father. I couldn't see it any other way. In time, I came to accept it as I did some of the other inexplicable facets of Appa's life. I now see the fact of Appa starting his day by adorning his forehead with vibhuti as not just a ritual, but an extension of that first act of initiation.

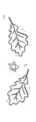

Meditation

Want to get something out of me? Forget the torture and the treats. A simple dark room and a ghost story will do. I am reduced to a shivering mass of fear when it comes to the dark and the supernatural that is associated with it. I have never seen a ghost or experienced anything paranormal but that doesn't deter my overactive imagination from conjuring up spirits that follow me in the dark or ghosts at the foot of my bed waiting for me to open my eyes. So, even after three decades of life on earth and raising kids of my own, I sleep with the night lamp on. I also cannot bear to listen to ghost stories, discuss the supernatural or watch a horror movie. In fact, I have watched every genre of film except horror.

Appa obviously has no such fears. In fact, he enjoys the dark. From as long back as I can remember, he would come back from work, have a bath and spend some time in a dimly lit room. Not only was the room kept dark, there were mirrors on four sides, reflecting the play of shadows, making the room seem extremely frightening to my young eyes. Later I realized he was meditating in that room and once I was old enough, I asked him why the room was so dimly lit and why it had those mirrors and why he spent so much time there. Did it not get boring? Didn't dark and macabre thoughts intrude during the meditation? The other places of worship I had seen were loud and bright, filled with gold and brass.

Appa smiled. Looking back, I understand that smile, especially since both my boys have started asking me questions about my habits and beliefs. His answer still echoes in my heart.

'All my life, I dreamt of achieving something big. I struggled, worked hard and with dedication and finally I achieved what I wanted. Fortune, fame and more. But as I climbed the ladder, I noticed something. The higher I got, the lonelier I became. There were very few around me who genuinely liked me. Many were jealous, which is a common human trait, but they turned that jealousy into an irrational hatred. My friends couldn't relate with me any more as my goals had changed and become more complex, as had the subjects that interested me, the problems that troubled me. Some people see loneliness at the top as security, but the reluctance of most people to have even a decent conversation with me troubled me. Most kept their distance due to respect, or a perceived difference in status. Alone in a constant crowd of people, I did not have time for anybody, not friends, not family, not even my own children. They were away at school when I left for work and fast asleep when I returned. Above all, I did not have time for myself.

'So every day, I carve out a bit of quiet time in that room. I am an actor who is constantly in the spotlight, literally and figuratively. The shooting lights are so bright that sometimes they hurt the eyes. [Remember, this was the late eighties.] So I keep the room dim to give my eyes some rest and I also feel hidden from the spotlight and at ease with myself. There's nobody to judge me, evaluate my actions or watch my every move. I can see myself in the mirror dimly, reflecting not just me but what has

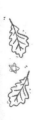

happened to me in the course of the day. The rights and wrongs I have done, or could have done, and in turn, what people have done to me. Have I used the day that god has given me well? Did I deserve it? What have I learned from it? I reflect on all this and absorb the lessons that are revealed in return.

'Each of the four mirrors gives me an illusion of being outside myself and hence outside the issue I am thinking about. It gives me a different perspective, sometimes four different perspectives. I have always been of the opinion that everything should be analysed and thought through from different angles before any conclusions are arrived at, or decisions made, and the mirrors are a physical manifestation of those different perspectives. The room is my homework. It helps me deal with my isolation and the loss of perspective that it brings. It comforts me and it is my alone time. I need it to analyse whether I am growing or stagnating, because at the top, nobody tells you that. Everybody should have this "me" time to sit back, outside your everyday life, and see how you have weathered the precious twenty-four hours that god has given you. I am a clean slate again when I step out of the room. I am ready to sleep well and face the next day. It has now become a duty that I owe to my own well-being. I grow there and I learn there.'

Mirrors have never been the same for me again. I now try to see not just my outer reflection, but also my inner self and try and find the strength to always remain true to myself. Because whatever happens, I cannot hide from the reflection in the mirror. From myself.

I was fascinated by my father's philosophy and for the most part, I have tried and tested it in my own life. As for my fear of the unknown, Appa always says, if there is good in the world, there has to be bad for balance to be maintained. Think dark thoughts and fear will surround you. Think good thoughts and good will come to you. Which is easier said than done, so my night lamp still stays on.

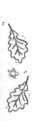

The Lord

A whole generation of Indian women consider their husbands to be their lord and master. Not my mother. For her, Tirupati Lord Venkateswara is the be-all and end-all, though Appa comes a very close second and is almost on the same pedestal. So here is the one story that I never tire of hearing and I can watch any number of repeat shows of my mother narrating it.

Once upon a time there was a middle-class, college-going girl in Chennai, studying English literature at Ethiraj College for Women. She was not like other girls of her age. She wanted to dedicate her life to social causes. Her other great love was music. So, at an early age, she decided marriage was not for her. Her parents worried about this, but she was happy with her life. Destiny, though, had other plans for her.

One day, the girl's sister convinced her to go along and watch a movie at the local theatre. A man appeared on the screen and her steadfast young mind was disturbed for the first time. She felt a strange connection to this tall, dark hero, who was unlike any other actor. It burned at the back of her mind. Fate too had seen the connection. Not long after, she was asked to interview an actor for the college magazine. Her elder sister's husband was part of the movie industry. He got her an interview with none other than that charismatic hero, the one who had disturbed the quiet of her mind. In the span of one interview, a soulmate was discovered. Like in the script of a blockbuster, the superhero fell for the simple college girl with high ideals. And in true Tamil movie style, he told her (not asked her) at their first meeting, 'I will marry you' and the girl surrendered, like a devotee might before a favourite deity.

That was not the end of the fairy tale. The families agreed and a wedding date was fixed. The hero was one of the trustees of the Tirumala Tirupathi Devasthanam while Sri N.T. Rama Rao was the chief minister. (He stepped down after his term was over.) Hence they were allowed to worship at the sanctum sanctorum. In his humility, the hero never misused his position. He considered himself to be just another ardent devotee and was surprised to discover that his fiancée shared the same devotion.

At the sanctum sanctorum of the Lord's abode, the hero took out the sacred tali and tied it around Amma's neck and they were joined as one. No pomp, no splendour, no time spent in long rituals and no stopping the stream of other eagerly waiting devotees. As far as I know, it is the only wedding to have been solemnized so close to the Lord. It was the perfect spiritual union.

I still get goosebumps imagining the scene. Appa's intensity and my mother's joy. Of course, according to me, the best part of the story comes later, when they were blessed with two bundles of joy, one after the other.

The newly-weds had a grand reception when they got back to Chennai, where the great NTR was a guest. Appa went up to him and thanked him for the privilege of having got married in front of Lord Balaji. NTR, with his characteristic grace, replied, 'I did not choose to do it, Lord Venkateswara did.'

The Lord of the Seven Hills has continued to grace my mother's devotion. Every devotee of his must have a story that demonstrates his love—problems averted, miraculous darshans and much more. My mother also has one. Eighteen years after the wedding, when she was on a pilgrimage to Tirupati, she reached the temple very late in the evening. She was travelling alone and back then, there were no late-night darshans, so she was feeling pretty disheartened. She walked in anyway, hoping to have a glimpse of the Lord before they shut, but the person guarding the queue complex told her to turn back.

She stood there alone, knowing that she had an urgent appointment the next day and would have to return the same night. The disappointment was immense. To come all this way and return without seeing Lord Balaji was almost a physical blow. She stood there praying, 'I have come to see you, I know I am late, but if you wish, please make it happen.'

The head priest was rushing for the closing of the sanctum. He saw Amma standing there alone in the empty temple courtyard, praying. 'What are you doing here so late, Amma? Come, let's go in and catch a glimpse before they close the doors,' he said. He led her to the temple. She was awestruck by her luck. The priest had not recognized her. He was just being solicitous to a desperate devotee. The Lord stood there glowing in the dark, as if waiting for her. Those who have seen the splendour of the eight-foot deity can imagine the scene. She fell at his feet, all else forgotten. Spellbound, not even remembering the prayers she had to say or the problems she wanted to leave at his feet. Then, remembering her surroundings, she got up to leave so that she would not delay the closing procedures. That was when the chief priest came by again.

'Amma, I have a request. We count the hundial collections at night and need a witness to sign the ledger at the end of the day. The person who usually does it has not been able to make it. Would it be possible to wait for a while and witness the total for us?'

Amma was dumbstruck at her luck. The priest was asking her to bask in her Lord's glow for some more time. She nodded and continued to stand there, gazing at the deity's visage, overwhelmed and filled with wonder. When the counting was done, Amma signed and crosschecked the locks and the amount. In her ecstasy, she did not realize she had made history. There were no other women witnesses in that temple ledger.

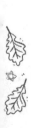

A Matter of a Thousand

Imagine a crisp thousand-rupee note, pink and fresh. A few years ago, it could buy a whole lot of things. Today—not so much. You may even have a couple of them in your wallet right now.

And don't bother denying it, that's what almost all of us want a lot more of. From the factory worker who wishes for a few thousand more to buy a bike, to a bank manager who wants a few more lakhs so he can afford to move to a better house, to the hot entrepreneur looking for a few million more to be invested in his company.

But what is the real value of a thousand rupees? To those with a background in economics or banking or commerce, who have figures and formulae running through their heads: Stop! That's not where I am headed.

My father was eleven years old when it happened. My eldest uncle was engaged to a girl from Somarhalli, which is a couple of hours by road from Bangalore. The engagement was conducted in the traditional way. The two families met, exchanged sweets and clothes, and agreed on a date. The year was 1961.

The wedding was to be held at the girl's place and two days before the date, the entire family was packed and ready. My grandfather's contribution to the wedding was to be a thousand rupees, to be given on the day of the wedding. He had mortgaged his 1200 sq. ft house to get the money, which was to be delivered to the house at 9 a.m., on the day they were supposed to leave. The scary part of this was that my grandfather did not have any supporting documents or a receipt for the mortgage. It was done entirely on trust.

Nobody came at 9 a.m. There was still no sign of the money at 2 p.m. Panic mounted, yet there was nothing to be done. There was no other way to get that kind of money, and no way to contact the moneylender. Remember, this was long before the era of telephonic communication. Appa recalls the tension building inside that small home. Ten family members waited, praying and hoping. Finally, every other activity came to a standstill and they all sat, every eye turned to the open door. No one said a word. My grandfather's face reflected their anxiety and the potential embarrassment, the shame the groom's family would face if they did not come up with the promised money.

Appa remembers being hungry but too scared to ask for food, and watching the female members of his family weep silent tears as the men sat around, staring at the door. The day passed and the night brought a thunderstorm with it. The door was shut, but every eye was still turned to it. The heavy silence was broken only by the sound of the rain and the thunder. Nobody ate, nobody spoke. Anxiety had turned to fear. My grandfather's face had turned to stone, but his eyes still watched the door, his lips moving silently in prayer. The storm was getting worse, the wind wailed outside and rainwater leaked through the roof. Nobody slept.

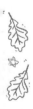

At 3 a.m., there was a knock on the door. At first Appa couldn't believe it. But the knock sounded again.

The entire household surged towards the door. There stood a man, barely holding on to a battered umbrella that was being thrashed around by the storm. Appa remembers thinking that at that moment, the man was like a god who had answered all their prayers.

The man stepped inside, dripping water, and pulled out a stack of old notes, which he handed over to my grandfather, while apologizing for the delay. Appa recalls the relief and the happiness on his father's face. And the thousand rupees that were responsible for this.

The family immediately left for the bride's place where the wedding was conducted simply but beautifully, and my aunt was brought home.

Invariably, every time I see a thousand-rupee note, I am reminded of this incident. Specifically, the deep emotion with which my father narrated it. It brought home to me the blessings I had, and I hope to pass this on to my sons. Their superstar grandfather learned the value of money the hard way, and his example will help them learn it with as little heartache as possible.

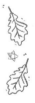

Fathers and Daughters

It was a few days before my eighteenth birthday. The magical day when the portals of adulthood would open and I would be free. (Don't fall off your chairs laughing; I was a pretty naïve seventeen-year-old.) There was some additional history to my birthday obsession. I was born on the first of January, which meant my special day was squeezed between roaring parties (which I was never ever allowed to attend), hangovers, making resolutions, temple visits, meditation and whatever else people do on New Year's day. I am not exaggerating. Unless you share my birthday, you cannot know the frustration of sharing your day with a global celebration, in which one half of the population is out celebrating and the other half is looking inward and praying.

'Happy New Year! Happy New Year! Oh, and by the way, happy birthday.'

So I had grand plans and high hopes for my eighteenth, the day I could legally drive, vote, drink and marry, but like all teenagers, I found something much more important to desire—I wanted to go to a club. An exciting new one had opened in orthodox Madras, and its wonders had reached even my sheltered ears. I just wanted to see what it was like inside one; drinking or dancing with strangers did not even cross my mind. A club symbolized every kind of freedom that being an adult would bring, but I had

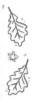

29

to overcome a huge hurdle. My Appa. Amma was protective, but then, mothers know when their daughters have grown up. As every woman knows, fathers have a peculiar idea about what their girls should do, or not do, irrespective of how old they are. My father was no different. I was, and will always be, his little girl. He himself had a rather conservative upbringing, and there was a strict line my sister and I could not cross. At the same time, he often surprised us with his adaptability to change when it came to our wishes, and keeping that in mind, I decided to ask him.

Now the smart ones reading this may ask a simple question. Why didn't I sneak out? With a strict family, in an orthodox city with friends and relatives around, it is difficult. But with a superstar as your father, in a city that worships him, under the watchful gaze of a pretty nosy society, it is impossible. To put it into perspective—I managed to have exactly one sleepover in the entire time I lived with my parents.

Since sneaking out was not an option, I came up with a brilliant plan. I would do the opposite and be entirely truthful about my birthday wishes. Appa has always appreciated honesty; besides, I was going to hit the big eighteen! So the day before the big one, I gathered up all my courage and asked him, 'Can I go to the new discotheque with my friends?' Appa froze for a minute before speaking. And his response stunned me.

'Of course, Kanna, good you brought it up. I will take you myself tomorrow!'

It was my turn to freeze. This was somehow worse than an outright no. But beggars can't be choosers. If it was my fate to go to my first club hangout with my father, so be it. Nothing could dampen the excitement of getting my way. I called up every one of my friends. I was going to party!

New Year's Eve, and all my wishes were coming true. A few

relatives and friends gathered at home and the mood was festive. I kept waiting for Appa to give the signal to leave. Nothing happened. I could not gather the courage to remind him. Every bit of it had gone into asking him for permission in the first place. Finally, at 11.30 p.m., when I had almost given up hope, my cousin came running up to me. 'Guess what! We are going to the club with your father.'

I almost burst with happiness.

My poor sister was bundled off to an aunt because she was underage and after gathering the rest of the family and friends, we left for the hotel in eight cars. Yes, eight cars. I know of couples who went on their honeymoon by bus, with their entire extended family, so this was tame in comparison. I sat next to Appa, grinning all the way.

The hotel was not prepared for the invasion of the Rajinikanth family. News spread and people started fighting to get into the place. Twenty bouncers were arranged. The police had to be called. It was turning into a pretty memorable birthday eve. The disco was electrifying: there was noise, colour, music and revelry in true New Year's eve style, heightened by the excitement of a star's presence in the middle of it all. I was overwhelmed. Though the bouncers formed a protective circle around us, people were crowding in, hoping to touch Appa, wish him, or just soak in the atmosphere around him. For someone brought up in relatively sheltered ways, it was awesome!

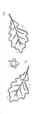

We had been in the club for all of ten minutes when it struck midnight. The entire family was enjoying themselves. Appa gave me a hug. 'Happy birthday, Kanna... happy?' I was ecstatic. Everyone around us was screaming Happy New Year, including the extremely loud DJ. But my father had wished me Happy Birthday first. I was on cloud nine.

The fall back was not very comfortable.

'Shall we leave?'

I thought I had heard him wrong. The confusion must have shown on my face.

'You wanted to see a discotheque, I have done my duty and shown you one. Let's leave now.'

Disappointment nearly brought tears to my eyes. I wanted to soak in the noise and excitement some more. Maybe dance with my cousins.

He gestured to Amma, who gathered us together, ready to leave. The crowd, by now, had become almost unmanageable. We left immediately and went home to sleep like good children. What an anticlimax for an eighteenth birthday. But looking back, I think it was the best fifteen-minute birthday party I have ever had.

I can sympathize with my father now and laugh at my younger self. He had to straddle two worlds, the traditional one he was brought up in and the modern one his daughters were growing up in. I may be prejudiced as his daughter, but I think he handled it like a true superstar!

Lungi & the Louvre

We Indians are a nosy lot. Within the span of a train journey, we often find out everything about our fellow travellers including their birth star. But when it comes to celebrities, we are thankfully much less prying than in the West. I see photos of scared, confused and often angry star children being chased by photographers and thank my lucky stars that I had a relatively normal childhood. Like most kids, my summer holidays were spent at my maternal grandparents' home, a modest three-bedroom apartment in the middle of the then sedate and calm Bangalore. Kids from the entire building played together in the evenings and friendships were formed. The ties forged then are strong even today. My grandmother believed in pampering her grandchildren throughout the vacation and would cook us delicious meals, take us out for ice cream, movies and shopping. Some of my favourite memories include taking long walks inside the Indian Institute of Science (IISc) campus and playing for hours with the other kids in the building.

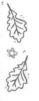

Thanks to my mother, vacations with Appa would also be somehow arranged. She understood their significance and convinced her workaholic husband of the importance of happy childhood memories that involved the entire family. So whenever possible, Appa would take some precious time off during our vacations and we would go on a holiday. Since he was instantly recognized everywhere in India, these holidays would often take us abroad, so that we could enjoy our time together as a normal family. We could go for walks and take him shopping like normal fathers and daughters.

One of these rare holidays was in Western Europe—London, Zurich, Bern and Paris—with a big group of family and friends. As usual my sister and I spent the entire flight watching movies back to back while Appa slept. I have always admired his talent for sleeping whenever he could, without being disturbed by anything that goes on around him. Back then I would wonder how he managed to keep so calm during the excitement of flying. Now I understand and sympathize. When I travel with the boys, I can't wait for them to settle down so I can take a much needed nap!

The next few days were fun and everyone was enjoying themselves immensely. There were around thirty suitcases and assorted hand baggage to be taken care of as we hopped from one city to the next. Inevitably, by the time we reached our beautiful Paris hotel overlooking the Eiffel Tower, one suitcase was lost and it was mine. The bellboy had delivered everyone's 'bursting at the seams' suitcases except mine. I had been so engrossed in the view that I forgot to check if my suitcase had arrived. I was sharing a room with my sister and cousin, who were so busy checking out the French menu and the foreign channels on TV that they just assumed everything had been delivered.

It was around noon and the plan was to leave the hotel as soon as everyone had freshened up, to see the sights. My sister went first, and once she was in the bathroom, I decided to unpack but couldn't find my suitcase. I ran out and checked every room that our family were in but there was no sign of it. The bellboy couldn't remember if mine was amidst the rest of the luggage and the front desk wasn't helpful at all. I walked around the hotel frantically looking for my black suitcase with the pink ribbons I had tied around the handle so that I could identify it easily. Giving up, I barged into my parents' room and flung myself on the bed, crying. I was in the city where fashion was foremost and didn't have any clothes to wear! Amma called the airport, the concierge and everyone in between, but no luck. By then everyone was ready to head out to lunch. I was dressed in smelly, wrinkled clothes and desperately needed to shower. There was no way I could borrow someone else's clothes either. My sister was much smaller than me, so were my cousins. (Okay, I will admit it, I was pretty big in my childhood.) My mother's and aunts' clothes were too large. They would fall off me.

I was crying helplessly on the bed when Appa came back into the room. 'Get up and go shower,' he said. 'You can wear my t-shirt and my lungi. It will look fine, trust me.'

Yes, my 'comfort first' Appa travelled with a lungi to Paris and was now ready to make it, and his chubby, image-obsessed tween, worthy of the fashion capital.

Styled by the stylish superstar and with his encouraging words, 'We are in Paris, let's make a statement!' ringing in my ears, I walked out more confident than I would have been in my own tee and jeans and feeling infinitely more special. I admit my memory of that day has 'style style dhan' as the background score! (Though I did have to put up with my sister teasing me until I bought new clothes. But then, it is the duty of the younger sister to bring the elder one back to earth, once in a while.)

Sisters

I enjoy having a sister. My very first memories of Soundarya, or Mittu as she is called at home, are of her visits to Bangalore. She would usually land up during my vacation time. She was a really cute, chubby baby and I loved her. She was also a total mommy's girl and would cling to Amma and want her around all the time. I always looked forward to their visits. It was almost a celebration at home—until I realized I had to share my toys with her! I wasn't used to sharing anything with anyone at that point. Little did I know that in a few years we would be inseparable and sharing a bedroom.

My sister and I are opposites in every sense. I grew up in a traditional household with my grandparents who had certain rules that had to be followed. She grew up with my mother who can never be anything but indulgent. I love classical dance and played the veena when I was growing up. My sister loved golf and played the piano. I am a voracious reader while she hardly reads books, but she can sketch well. I write and she is an artist. She is an extrovert, I am an introvert. She makes bold choices while I go with the flow. And there is just one difference that bothers me. We were both plump little babies, but after a point she lost all the baby weight and has remained stick thin!

Other than being related by blood, my sister and I share a special bond. It may have been created due to the circumstances of our birth and upbringing or the fact that Appa always gave a lot of importance to family. Family comes first and we both believe in that implicitly. No matter what happens, she will have my back and I hers. We aren't very demonstrative or clingy as siblings. I was never one to share my feelings openly; she understood that part of me and always worked around it. I treasure this non-judgemental aspect of our relationship and when we get an opportunity to let our hair down and enjoy ourselves, it has always been epic. Our most special moments have been unplanned, often ending in long gossip and bonding sessions that last through the night.

I sometimes do feel a little guilty about getting married and leaving home at twenty-two. She was younger and it would have helped to have an elder sister around. Instead, I jumped headlong into married life and all that it entails. She is much more emotional than I am and it took her some time to get used to my absence, though I do feel it made her stronger.

From a very young age, Soundarya was ambitious. She knew exactly what she wanted. While I wanted to marry and 'settle down', she wanted to become an entrepreneur. My choices have always been pretty conventional, whereas hers are bold. She went to Australia and learned graphic design much before it became a rage. When she got an opportunity to work with my father, 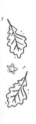 she cast him in a role that no other artist in India had been cast in before. I saw the fighter in her during the process of making *Kochadaiyaan*. It was the first of its kind in India and getting it off the ground was very difficult, involving new technology, software and equipment. Recreating the ideas that were revolutionary on paper into reality, that too in the motion capture format, was immensely challenging. I knew very little of the technology and saw the struggle only from the sidelines. She was doing something very different, but it was way ahead of its time. Amma was a huge pillar of support during those trying times. In fact I see a lot of Amma in Soundarya. There were several occasions when she could have shelved the work and walked away, but she saw it through and I admire her for that.

Though we both tell stories with our movies, mine tend to be raw, based in reality, and minimalist. My sister's canvas is larger than life and visually dramatic. And now, when we are collaborating on projects, it's both interesting and challenging. There is a comfort level and understanding which comes with being family, a certain informality that helps the creative process. We also know each other's strengths and weaknesses, and know how to work with, or around, them. At the same time, there are some lines that have to be drawn when it comes to doing any work in a professional environment and those lines are tougher to define when it comes to family.

Where our differences allow us to create a perfect balance is in our children's lives. Between us, we are now mothers to three boys who create pandemonium whenever they are together. Soundarya is a control freak when it comes to parenting. I am a stickler in certain matters but give a lot more freedom to the boys and between us we manage to create some semblance of discipline, much to Amma's amusement. Soundarya's son, Ved, the youngest among the boys, is the one who rules us all right now. His word is command.

Life hasn't always been easy, as it never is, but it has been a huge comfort to have a sister to share the experience. There is so much expected of us and there is only so much we can do, and I am thankful for the fact that there is one other person who understands this as well as I do. Mittu and I have lived with the limelight, the pressures and the challenges and come out of it stronger and closer.

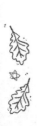

Bangalore Days

The best part of my childhood was spent with my maternal grandparents. This is not in any way meant to put my parents down, but anybody who has had loving grandparents knows how special they can be. If parents are a sustaining meal, grandparents are the much looked forward to dessert!

My grandparents were a perfect mix of the traditional and the modern. They loved visiting temples and they loved their evening get-togethers with friends coming over for drinks, dinner and a rousing game of checkers. They were staunch Brahmin vegetarians, but they enjoyed their buns and cakes made with eggs. They enjoyed music and movies. Both loved a good argument and laughed at the silliest of jokes cracked by the other. Grandmother was the agony aunt of the street. Women on their way to office would stop by for a scoop of her famous bisibele bath to perk up their lunchboxes. Three of her friends would inevitably turn up after their siesta for coffee and murukku. Teachers and even nuns from my school, which was just across the street, came in sometimes to say hello. I even remember a teenaged boy from a street away complaining about the constant arguments he had with his mother over late nights out while my grandmother served him snacks. In short, my grandmother had a way with people. Including me.

One of her friends was a shopkeeper with a fancy store that was famous in our area. I would pester her to take me there and ask for almost everything in the shop and somehow come back home with just a candy, yet not be upset in any way. My grandparents were happy with their simple life and enjoyed what they had to the fullest. I am not saying they had perfect lives (although I hope they did) but that they never showed anything but grace and zest for life when I was around.

I wish we as parents could do things as effortlessly as they seemed to. I have seen children exposed to the bitterness of the adults around them and wondered what scars it would leave. I have seen adults who still grapple with issues from their childhood.

Since my school in Bangalore was just across the road from home, I would occasionally walk over with my grandmother. She was a bold woman who could strike up a conversation with anybody. She admired women who worked outside the home, and would point them out to me. Women who had a sense of their own worth and did not depend on the men around them for it. Though she lent a sympathetic ear to just about everybody, she had no time for women who felt sorry for themselves or complained without doing anything about it. I remember her telling a particularly whiny woman to 'buck up, stand on your feet and stop sitting around crying about things that you cannot change'.

We used to travel to Chennai quite often and once we saw a lady pilot. My grandmother went on and on throughout the flight about how wonderful she looked and what a great example she was for young girls like me. She didn't stop there; she wondered aloud how I would look in a pilot's uniform. Once, we watched a movie about a daring woman lawyer, portrayed by one of the leading actresses of the day. She immediately started talking about how happy she would be if someday, I were to become a lawyer and argue a case and win people's hearts. This happened every time she saw a woman who had a career other than that of a homemaker. I got used to it and over time realized that she was drilling it into me for a reason. Her daughters, despite their liberal upbringing, had ended up choosing not to work. I think she missed seeing her daughters becoming successful in their own right in a profession she admired, like law or medicine. In her own generation, it had been next to impossible. So she directed her wishes towards me. She would speak about how one day I would find the zeal and the willpower to prove myself, to become an independent woman who could stand strong on her own, yet care for her loved ones. About how she would burst with pride when she saw me in that position. As I grew a little older, I was very attracted to the law as a profession. Fuelled by movies and myths, I would daydream about arguing brilliantly in court while my grandmother looked on proudly. I would imagine the judge's reaction, the cruel opposition lawyer, and the poor accused woman. I guess I was of a directorial bent even then, though my head was filled with every movie cliché in the book.

My grandfather was a fountain of information and I would ask him a hundred questions about being a lawyer. The ochre red structure of the High Court fuelled my imagination even further. I spoke about it nonstop and my grandmother would beam with happiness. I think she was already imagining me in a lawyer's robe. Little did I know how much pain these childish ambitions would cause me someday.

When I was around nine, I came back to Madras. The move was heart-wrenching. I loved Bangalore and living with my grandparents. The apartment, the morning walks, the crowd of friends. Appa and Amma would visit very often, and I visited them, but my anchor was in Bangalore.

Sometime before the move, my grandfather had started explaining to me how big a star Appa was. I used to watch his movies with my grandmother and the next time I saw him, we would discuss it avidly. My grandfather later told me these 'avid discussions' usually involved me explaining the whole movie to him from my perspective and him listening in amused silence. He also told me that the day my parents left, I would be strangely sad. I didn't want to leave Bangalore, but at the same time, I did not want them to leave. It was a weird emotion. I would cry as they left, but at the same time, refuse their offer of taking me home with them. I was one confused kid!

It was a movie of Appa's that changed things around. I do not recall which one, but it had a scene where the villain dramatically stabs him. I was old enough to know movies are not real, but this scene affected me like no other. I burst out crying. My grandmother recalls that I wanted to talk to Appa immediately and wouldn't stop crying until he spoke to me over the phone and consoled me. That night I had nightmares. I mumbled for Appa in my sleep. My grandparents were greatly disturbed by my behaviour.

When I was first brought to them, it was because of concerns about my mother's health. She couldn't take care of two children by herself after my sister was born and deal with her health issues at the same time. My grandparents were more than happy to look after me. By then all their children had flown the coop and they were lonely in their empty nest, so I was a welcome relief.

Even after Amma recovered, I continued to stay with them since both of us were happy with the arrangement. This incident, though, made them feel selfish. They felt they were keeping me

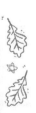

away from my parents and it was something I would regret later. A week went by and my grandfather was so distraught that he didn't go to work for the entire duration. Finally they realized that they had to let me go. Arrangements were made for me to leave for Chennai and live with my parents.

I didn't realize the significance of that last trip. It was a usual Chennai visit for me. They knew I would make a fuss, so they behaved as they normally did.

I was left at home and though my grandparents came to visit very frequently, it was not the same. I was used to being the centre of attention, but now I had to deal with an entirely new and busy household. I had a room to myself at my grandparents', now I had to share with my sister. A new school, new friends, and a new routine. My parents were very happy to have me back. Amma was constantly smiling and Appa loved coming home to both his daughters. I slowly realized this was for the best, but I never forgot the love my grandparents had for me. My love for everything related to law was also their legacy, though it would come to haunt me later in my life. But that is another story for another chapter.

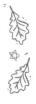

The Law of Losses

The move from Bangalore to Madras was traumatic. I cried every day. My grandparents would come rushing over and even stay for a while, but they refused to take me back. Appa was doing around five movies a year and that meant extended periods away from home. Amma had to divide her time between my sister and me. She couldn't let me go back. I now understand how much she must have hated sending me away and how my choice of staying with my grandparents must have hurt the very core of her being. She tried her best, and one of the ways she got my mind off things was by allowing me to join classes that would keep me busy. I joined veena, tennis, classical dancing and music classes. I settled in after a few months and started enjoying the new activities and the new school. The only thing that didn't change was my ambition to become a lawyer. I even dressed up as one for the school fancy-dress competition.

Towards the end of my middle-school, Amma started a school called Ashram. She had always been interested in teaching. When my sister and I came home from school, she would review the day's work and teach us using a small blackboard with a line drawn in the middle. One side was for me and one for my sister, which my sister would forget immediately and end up confusing with my work, which would finally result in her having

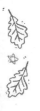

to do hers afresh. Amma's methods were always fun, with easy shortcuts to remember dates, concepts, etc. She never liked the idea of rote learning and encouraged us to learn at our own pace and reproduce material as we had understood it. The ranking system also upset her. She believed that giving grades was better for children and that each child was unique. I think she realized the lack of good schools at that point and decided to start one herself, where these theories could be put into practice.

Ashram became one of the best-known schools in the city, but back then there was a lot of confusion as to whether I should join the new school or stay in the prestigious school that I was already studying in. Finally it was decided that my sister and I would move. How would it appear if the children of the founder did not study in the school? Another adjustment period was in store for me.

The school started off small, with the intention of evolving a different way of learning. It was a revolutionary idea at a time when people were scrambling around for admission to conventional schools and trying to make their children either doctors or engineers. I was in the first batch and the school grew with me. From a school with thirty students in each class, I moved to a batch of twenty students in all. My life turned into a tiny circle of school and home, both overseen by my mother. People assume that I had it easy, but it was just the opposite. Amma made sure that my sister and I weren't treated any different from the other students. In fact we were expected to be model students and behave perfectly. The teachers also made sure they didn't say or do anything that could be misconstrued as favouritism. Not only that, they would talk about every move we made to Amma. I wouldn't call it a complete loss of privacy, but it came close to that. She thought it was best for us and after a while I got used to it. There was one lovely, soft-spoken teacher who stood out. She taught us English and I studied hard for her lessons and scored well. I hated science, even though Ashram had a policy of teaching through application. Being the first batch at any school has its disadvantages and advantages and I still wonder what it would have been like, had I remained in my previous school. As they say, the grass is always greener on the other side.

Amma was always overprotective of us. I think circumstances made her so. The fact that I had been away from her for the initial part of my childhood may have contributed to the possessiveness. She once told Appa that she would look for grooms for us, who would agree to stay with the girl's parents. Appa laughed at that. I still had ambitions of being a lawyer; everybody would encourage me except Amma, who would remain silent whenever the topic came up.

As school drew to a close, I started preparations for the law entrance exams and to apply to colleges across the country. Amma was against it. She wanted me to stay at home. She tried talking me out of it, but I was adamant. Arguments and rows became very common. One night, as I was studying, she came and sat next to me, watching me. I found it very odd and asked her what the matter was. She said she would like to sit with me for some time. I nodded my head in agreement and soon realized it was comforting to be around my mother without fighting or trying to win an argument. Then, after a while, she softly asked me if she could speak. I nodded again. She said, 'I do not want you to leave town to study anywhere else in India or abroad. I prefer to be safe than sorry. I have a responsibility to your father to bring you up safely and I don't think I can do that when you are not with me. We will find out if there is any way you can study from home or if I can extend the school to include higher education too.'

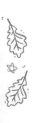

She then told me not to bother my father about any of this, and left.

I must admit I didn't understand her point of view at all. So many of her own friends had sent their children abroad to study and seemed proud of their ambitions. But my mother didn't want me to leave the nest at all. I wanted to ask Appa to intervene, but was confused by her instruction to not talk to him about it. For those of you who do not understand my hesitation, you have to remember that Appa was unbelievably busy during our childhood and the responsibility of bringing us up lay with my mother. When we were children, Amma instructed us carefully before letting us speak with Appa. She wanted his rare evenings at home to be stress free. I am sure she meant well. She didn't want Appa to hurt us by word or deed if we got boisterous. (Which we did very often at other times.) This doesn't mean he was always tense and grumpy and needed his wife to police the children. He was always pleasant at home and Amma's insistence on good manners ensured that we had quality time with him.

A few days later Amma and I reached a compromise. I would write one entrance exam for a reputed law school that had limited seats and if I got through, we would take it from there. I went to a good college close to home for six months while studying for the exams. She was sure I wouldn't get through; I was determined to do my best. I wrote the exam and I got through. I was over the moon. My dreams were finally coming true. I told Appa, who was very happy for me, though I think he didn't actually know what I had gone through or the magnitude of what I had achieved. Amma hugged me when I gave her the news and I waited to hear what she had to say.

When she did speak, it was like someone had stabbed me in the gut. It was a residential collage, she said, so it would be impossible for me to go. She had talked to a few people to see if I could be exempted from staying on campus, but it was in vain. I told Appa how much it meant to me, I wanted him to enquire about the place, to see that it was a big deal and also to prove that it was safe. He did, and tried to convince Amma, but she wouldn't budge. Her daughter could not stay by herself, away from the family, however reputed the school was.

I stopped going to college and sat at home. If I wasn't going to be a lawyer, I didn't want to study any more. Amma, in her own way, tried to make amends. She ran from pillar to post and somehow managed to get permission to start a diploma course in her own institution. The system isn't easy and a lot of protocol, not to mention investment, is involved, but she managed to do it all and also brought in the best teachers she could find.

I earned that diploma in legal studies, but it wasn't the real thing. And yet, when you are young, you bounce back pretty quickly. I moved on, although once in a while, when things got rough, I would bring it up just to rile Amma.

Then life happened, I got married, and my interest in movies grew. I accompanied Dhanush on shoots and watched different directors at work. I did not think of my early ambitions any more. Soon I became a mother and that overtook everything else in my life. I was a full-time mother and I enjoyed every minute of it. Of course there were sleepless nights and messy days, but it was all an adventure for me.

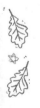

Once, when Yatra was a year old and I had a moment to rest from the child rearing, I was going through old photographs and saw one of the diploma award ceremony. I stared at it for a while, marvelling about how things change. Yet, the thought of how badly I had wanted it left an aftertaste that lingered for days after I saw that photo. I found myself searching for correspondence courses online. I wasn't very net savvy and may have missed something. But I was obsessed. There was no way I could attend college at this stage of my life, I knew I would find it more than a little embarrassing. I asked a few people and they hadn't heard of any law courses that could be done sitting at home. I didn't give up, I called everyone I knew who was connected with the law. A very close family friend finally came up with a plan. She spoke to the head of a law school that was located a couple of hours away from Chennai. He would let me study at home, he said, but I would have to come to the college to write the exams every term and attend any relevant practical classes. I hugged my friend tight and after digging out all my certificates, enrolled for that year's course. The college accepted my application. Dhanush and Appa were very excited for me. I was on cloud nine. My husband had also missed out on college and was happy that I could do it.

Now came the tough part. How could I study without the support of teachers? It had been years since I passed out of school. I wondered if I could write a single lucid paragraph without help. A cousin came to my rescue. She had just started classes at the city's premier law college. She responded to my SOS call and agreed to play tuition teacher. The next step was to find time for it all. My young one had started playschool, so I had a couple of hours then; the rest of the studying happened when he was asleep. But getting back to academics was tougher than I had imagined. I would sit down to study but household chores, my son, other work that I had, everything crowded into my head, leaving little room for theories or case studies. When my cousin arrived to teach me, I would be all enthusiasm and excitement, but once she started, I would begin to yawn. It was weird. My eyes would droop, but once the class was over, I would be as bright as day. Concentrating after being away from studies for so long was extremely tough. But I refused to give up and plodded on. Dhanush would find my yawning and cribbing extremely funny. He would shake his head as I drooped through the classes and then at night as I struggled with the notes I had taken. As the semester passed, I got the hang of it. My cousin was impressed with my progress from a blank-eyed, yawning student to one who could now answer questions. My son would come up to me and ask a hundred questions. He couldn't understand why I was studying at home and not at school with a proper teacher. He wanted to do the same thing. A pretty good excuse to miss playschool!

The semester came to a close and the day before the exams, I went home to get my parents' blessings. I had my notes for some last-minute revision, a new notepad and a pouch filled with new pens. These were placed in the puja room. I had to leave four hours ahead to reach the college in time. I was tense and called the poor principal at 10 p.m. He was very gracious and assured me that all arrangements had been made. Nobody knew except a few professors and they had strict instructions not to tell anyone.

I had a warm glass of milk and went to bed early, but I couldn't sleep. I am ashamed to say I had to take a sleeping pill. I woke up before dawn and found myself calm. I had a quick shower, a few moments in the puja room, then I kissed my sleeping son and left for college. Dawn broke along the way, as I looked through my notes. My phone pinged. Amma's was the first message of the day. It said, 'Do well'.

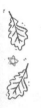

Appa called in a while and wished me well, and as I reached the gates of the college, Dhanush called too. I was feeling as ready as I could be. But when we entered the gates and I saw the buildings looming ahead, everything flew out of the window. I wanted to ask the driver to turn back home. I found a few staff members waiting for me and ridiculously asked them if I could write the exam in a room alone. The request was politely turned down. When I walked into the hall, I could hear a few gasps and murmurs. I wanted to dig a hole in the ground and disappear. The murmuring continued while I wondered why the exam wasn't starting. I felt like bolting home. Those late-night struggles, the effort I had made just to get here, to write this exam, stopped me. Thankfully, the teacher started handing out the sheets and everyone went quiet. She came close to me and smiled. 'Relax and just concentrate on your paper. I am sure you will do well.' Just as I felt a wave of relief, she continued, 'Once you are done, hand in the paper and please wait. The staff want to take a picture with you.'

I am sure she thought I was ill, because instantly the blood drained to my feet and I could barely breathe. There were almost a hundred people around me, staring at me. Panic gripped my insides, but I refused to give in. It wasn't anything new; I had been gawked at from an early age. I could handle it. Picturing my grandmother in my mind, I opened the question sheet and closed out everything else. Thankfully I knew the answers and it felt as though things were finally going my way. I finished and the thoughts came crowding back into my head. Would the other students think I was a spoilt brat for the concession I was getting? Did they assume the only reason I was here was due to my father's influence? Did they wonder if I had studied at all? Given the rampant corruption in our country, even if I passed, they might wonder if it was because of some additional help I had received.

I handed the paper over and almost ran to the car. The dean was standing outside and I had to thank him before leaving. The moment I shook hands with him and turned, there were around fifty cameras at the gate. Somehow, between the time I walked in and the time it took me to finish, the news had leaked and a contingent of press persons had arrived. The dean was as surprised as I was and kept trying to apologize. He was drowned out by the noise.

'How come you are here? What made you come here to study? How long have you been doing the course? What did your father have to say about it? What was your husband's reaction?'

I ran to my car and took off. The dean called me and apologized again. Nobody knew how the news had leaked. I told him it wasn't his fault. We both realized that my presence would be a disturbance for the rest of the students. There was no way I could continue with the course. I had to cut short my dreams again.

The poor dean also had his own troubles for a while after that. The press wouldn't leave him alone. They continued to stalk the college and its students, thinking that I would be back.

I must also mention that my stubbornness, subsequent marriage and moving out must have caused some change in Amma's thinking. That is the only way I can explain it. Soundarya was in school when I had fought to study outside Madras and she wasn't involved in any of the discussions or arguments. So she didn't realize the importance of what she eventually achieved. My sister wanted to pursue graphics and multimedia, it was her passion, and she applied to Australia with full support from my parents and got through. I am no saint and when she first burst into my room with the news, I was a little disconcerted. I was very happy for her, after all she is my sister and I wouldn't have wanted her to go through the same suffocating rigmarole that I went through. All I wanted to know was what had changed my mother's mind. I never get around to asking her, and then it

didn't matter. I had been blessed with a beautiful life and there was so much to look forward to.

I did not think of anything to do with studies for a long time after that. I had my second baby, directed movies, did some writing and became thoroughly busy. Between having the two boys, I had started dancing again. (It stopped again for a while after the second one.) Dhanush needed help with production and I took over. I was happy with the various roles I was playing and my earlier disappointments never crossed my mind.

A couple of years later, during a brainstorming session at work, the subject of law came up and I explained my fascination to a colleague. She wondered aloud why I didn't pursue it again. I told her I had too much on my plate and I felt that the universe just didn't want me to do it. I had tried and failed too many times. I enjoyed the subject but practising as a lawyer was not on my agenda any more. Movies had spun their magic on me.

A week later, as we were talking, she placed a few papers on my desk and asked me to take a look. I had not expected to see the crests of international universities and glossy brochures explaining options that someone at my stage of life could take advantage of. I was reluctant to go through the material. It lay on my table for a week. My colleague kept asking me to take a look and I resisted. Two weeks passed and one day, as I was checking my email, I came across an acceptance letter from a university abroad. It was for a four-year degree in criminology. I read it again and again, wondering why my name was on the letter. It turned out that my dear colleague had enrolled me in the course. I couldn't practise law, but I could study the subject, its ins and outs, even discover why it fascinated me so much. Criminology includes the psychology of crime and research into its prevention. I was hooked. The incident at the college had made me realize that I could never finish a proper law degree, with its emphasis on practice. This was the perfect alternative. My colleague had made me realize that it's never too late and when every door slams in your face, a window opens somewhere. All I needed was a nudge and thankfully someone had provided it.

When Dhanush came to know of the course, he was not surprised at all. He did exactly what he had done the previous time and supported me all the way. 'If it makes you happy, do it. Nobody in the family is going to judge you or be dismissive.' Dhanush has strong, educated women in his own family. Both his sisters are well-regarded doctors.

The thought of studying made me a little apprehensive. What inspired me at that moment was a family member. She had completed her PhD when she was eighty years old—I thought she was a rock star. I look in the mirror every day and draw inspiration from women like her, including the one who brought me up and now watches over me from somewhere above. As I work on my assignments, which are challenging but fun, my sons sit alongside and finish their homework. It is an inspiration for them too.

I believe that education is the greatest gift one can give to one's own self-worth. There is no satisfaction like it, especially if you are passionate about it.

The induction for my course was to be held at the college. It would be a four-day affair and I packed my bags with excitement and fear. The last time I had entered a college, it had been traumatic. These four days were to be filled with classes and lectures that would equip us to study from home.

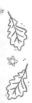

I landed and was driven to the university town. It was a very different experience for me. An entire town dedicated to a university, serving the students and the professors. By 7 p.m.

everything shut down. The town rose early and slept early. On the first day, I stepped out apprehensively. I had packed a satchel and felt like a real student, walking to my classes from the place I was staying in. Nobody looked and nobody stared. I got lost and had to muster up all my courage to ask the way from total strangers. It was the first time I was having to fend for myself. All the precautions drilled into my head about surrounding myself with the right people, about strangers taking advantage, crowded into my head. Should I make conversation? Should I smile? What if a conman followed me to the hotel? Paranoia gripped me. But I forced myself to remain calm and, slowly but surely, found my way.

The classes were a revelation. There were people from every walk of life, from every age group. I finally felt comfortable. The professor came in and we introduced ourselves. The entire class and the professor himself were shocked to learn that I had come all the way from India for the induction. Most of them were from cities and towns that were just a couple of hours' drive away. The first two days, I kept looking over my shoulder as I walked to class. I would wake up and look through the peephole several times in the night to make sure I was alone. But the following two days were fun. I learned to enjoy the experience without worrying about anything and I came back home feeling I had vanquished a monster that had nagged me all my life.

I fared quite well in my first year and am working towards finishing the degree. I intend to finish it this time. As they say, third time's the charm.

We Take It Black

Picture this—there are six steel tumblers on a tray. One contains coffee decoction, one has hot water, one has milk, and the rest are empty. The first tumbler is picked up and a bit of coffee decoction is poured into one of the empty tumblers. Then a little hot water is added and the consistency checked. This is repeated till found satisfactory. Then the milk is carefully poured into the mix of coffee and water, drop by drop, until the right consistency is attained. It does not stop there. This mixture is then strained into another empty tumbler. Finally, this watery, lukewarm, slightly milky concoction is poured into the sixth tumbler and sipped.

This is how Amma drinks her coffee, twice a day. Every day.

Coffee is an integral part of many people's lives. If we woke up one day and all the coffee on earth had disappeared, I think eighty per cent of the world would come to a standstill. The first thing to touch your lips in the morning, it's what runs meetings and conversations. 'Go for a coffee' has acquired connotations from 'I am interested in you' to 'we need to talk'.

My affair with coffee began very early. It was an important part of the routine in my grandmother's home. I woke up to the amazing smell of ground coffee as it mixed with steaming hot water in a filter that stood prominently in a nook near the kitchen window. It had once belonged to my great-grandmother and had been passed on to my grandmother. I would brush and wash quickly, then spend a few moments in the puja room before rushing to the kitchen for my glass of milk. My grandmother would be busy at the stove, which had a big vessel of boiling milk on it. Pots and pans would be strewn about and lunch bags and carriers sat on the counter waiting to be packed, for me to take to school and for my grandfather to take to work. On my arrival, she would pour a strong cup of filter coffee for herself and a big glass of milk for me. I used to nag her until she added a small dollop of coffee decoction into my warm milk. It made me feel all grown up and added a bit of dignity to the next item on my morning agenda—reading *The Hindu* aloud with my grandfather before heading to school. (I know children aren't supposed to have coffee, but back then it wasn't such a big deal and I haven't suffered any ill effects. The quantity was also quite negligible.)

My grandfather read the entire newspaper page by page every morning, but he had a quirky way of doing it. He would start at the sports section and head towards the main news. 'So that I can start with something positive and light, first thing in the morning' was his answer when I asked him about it. People dying, hurting each other, cheating or worse, could always wait till later in the morning. Thanks to my grandfather, that's how I read the paper too—back to front. (And now, since the advent of the supplement, that's what I reach for on most days.)

My grandparents were very health conscious and had a disciplined lifestyle. Early morning walks were indispensable and once I had become old enough, I had to accompany them at 5 a.m. every day. I think now that they did not want to leave me alone in the house while they went out, so this was the compromise. I am glad they took me. The IISc grounds were beautiful and

I was the only kid around, so I got a lot of attention. Later I noticed a father-and-son pair, the slightly chubby son pushed and prodded by the father into running with him. On weekends, my grandparents and four of their 'walking friends' would meet at a coffee shop on the main road just outside the institute gates and chat. A small cup of coffee would be poured out for me too. They would take turns cooling the hot, fragrant liquid before passing it on to my eager hands. As I grew up, the coffee I drank started to strongly resemble how my grandfather took it. When I came back to Madras, the coffee did not taste the same as it did at my grandmother's place. That was when she explained that the smallest of things can drastically change the taste of filter coffee. From the ratio of chicory in the coffee blend to any difference in the quality of water. The filter in each house is also different. So I discovered with great sadness that it was almost impossible to replicate the taste that I had loved so much. I went to the other extreme then, and took to instant coffee. It was quick and easy, and though it took a while to get used to the taste, convenience won. Every time my grandmother saw me drinking it, she would mutter angrily about how modern conveniences had taken over everything, including a simple cup of filter coffee.

How you like your coffee can be indicative of your character too. Appa likes his strong, with just a hint of sugar, and piping hot. It has to go from the stove to his lips; anything less than boiling hot is considered mediocre. I have already explained Amma's painstaking coffee ritual. The only time she couldn't follow it was when we were travelling and she was compelled to have instant coffee. When I reached my twenties, I became a little (a lot!) conscious of my weight and decided to do away with milk in my coffee. I used to have five to eight cups a day and eventually decided to do away with sugar too. Amma was

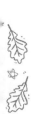

aghast. She constantly chided me, saying it was harmful to drink so much coffee, but do we ever listen to our mothers?

Once I got married, I discovered that my husband enjoyed his coffee the way I did. Black. He did add sugar though. Surprisingly we had never gotten around to having a coffee together during our courtship and he had no clue about my coffee addiction. During some conversation about coffee, it was my mother-in-law who told me how he came to like it black. Apparently his grandmother used to give them black coffee when they were kids and though all his siblings got over the habit and started adding milk when they grew up, he continued having his black. I was taken aback. I couldn't of course criticize her mother-in-law in front of her and I did not know the circumstances, but as soon as I could, I asked my husband why his grandmother gave black coffee to little children. I remembered how much flak my own grandmother got for putting a hint of coffee into my milk. Dhanush then told me that his grandmother had a bunch of kids to feed and no way to afford milk on a daily basis, so she would mix sugar in watery coffee that had a tinge of milk and give it to them. As he grew up, the quantity of milk reduced and black coffee became a habit. Listening to him, I was struck by the two extremely diverse ways in which we had both come to like our coffee black.

I have tried to reduce my intake of coffee and to add milk whenever I can; my husband continues to take his black. Amma hasn't changed her six-tumbler habit and Appa still loves his coffee strong and hot. My children don't drink coffee at all, but once in while I add a dollop to their milk from the filter from my childhood that has come down to me from my grandmother.

Festivals

Unity in diversity has taken a beating in recent times, but what most people forget is that living in India is unique because of the variety of cultures one gets to experience. The film fraternity, in particular, is known for its celebration of diversity, but something similar is also visible in homes across the country. Take my example. I was born into a Hindu family and for the first nine years of my life lived with my Brahmin grandparents, who sent me to a convent school in Bangalore run by Christian nuns. A typical morning for me involved getting ready and then walking into the puja room where my grandfather would be worshipping Lord Ganesha, Hanuman and Durga. There was a little brass bell that I would ring as he did the aarti with camphor flames and towering brass multi-tiered lamps.

The school was right across the road from my grandparents' home and on most days, my grandmother would stand on the balcony and watch, a prayer on her lips, until I disappeared into the school building. Then it was time for morning prayers at the school, where sometimes the younger kids were taken to the chapel. I don't remember feeling any sense of confusion. I just grew up with a healthy balance of Jesus and Hanuman.

I remember my grandmother making vada, murukku and tea for the teachers who often came to visit after school, not that I got any brownie points for that—in fact they went to great lengths to ensure they weren't in any way partial to me. My grandmother's chakkara pongal was also a great hit among my classmates from other communities. I, for my part, loved to taste the variety of snacks that other kids brought to school. Christmas was also a fun time; my grandmother and I would put up a tree and decorate it. A red star would be hung in the balcony and lit at night. Presents waited for me under the tree on Christmas morning.

The mix of cultures did not end there. Like many others from Madras, I was taken to the local dargah to be prayed over whenever I had a nightmare or was unwell. When I returned to Madras, I was admitted to a Hindu school, but Christmas was celebrated at home with great fervour. There was a spruce tree in our garden that would be beautifully decked up and on Christmas Eve we would drive from church to church, starting at the magnificent Santhome Basilica, admiring the beautiful lights, decorations and the strains of Christmas carols that sweetened the air. We would buy balloons and Santa Claus masks from roadside vendors and play with them well into the night. I still remember visiting a temple at that time, outside which a woman stood selling flowers. In her stall was a small Christmas tree decorated with flowers, with a small oil lamp flickering at its feet.

Eid was also something I looked forward to, mostly for the yummy biriyani, I must admit. One of Appa's friends used to send over a box of piping-hot biriyani every Eid for Appa. He knew my mother, sister and I were vegetarians, so he would send a vegetarian version as well. And he hasn't forgotten me even after I moved into my husband's house. Two generous portions of vegetable biryani are sent for Dhanush and me every year.

Appa's deep sense of spirituality also had a great influence on me. Although the rituals and cuisines were the chief attraction at the festivals, he never forgot to remind us of the underlying meaning of these. The sacrifice that is celebrated at the end of Ramzan, the message of love at Christmas and the triumph of good that is enacted at most Hindu festivals.

Amma, on the other hand, loved Janmashtami. It was her favourite god's birthday and was celebrated over three days. People came over for bhajans and puja. Little feet were drawn in rice batter and the marble idols of Krishna and Radha, which are my mother's pride and joy, were bathed and garlanded. She still offers prayers to them every day. When I moved into a home of my own, I wanted to continue celebrating these festivals so that my sons could also grow up understanding the beauty of different religions and communities. And I do take them to temples, churches and dargahs, even if they consider it a tad boring, more for my own peace of mind.

Choices

Even before the term 'foodie' became famous, or should I say infamous, I was in love with eating. Mealtimes during my childhood were special. We were lucky to have a string of wonderful cooks and each meal had a minimum of four to five dishes. That luck seems to have run out now. Good cooks are hard to find. My cook's whims and fancies plus the stress of diplomatically directing her to prepare better meals sometimes scare me more than directing a full-length film!

Although I loved variety when it came to food, Appa would help himself to only one dish, irrespective of the number of dishes placed before him. Due to the unreliable work timings that the film industry has, most of his meals were packed and sent from home. The few times he managed to make time from his hectic shooting schedule to have a meal with the family, he would carefully choose one dish and enjoy it thoroughly. I noticed this even when we went out to eat. He would have breads or rice with one accompanying dish and that was it. Rotis or rice with one curry, biriyani with raita, noodles with chicken... you get the picture. No nibbling on starters, no sampling of appetizers, no dipping into more than one side dish. Even the second helping would be the same simple choice as the first. As one who firmly believes that variety is the spice of life, particularly when it comes to food, I found this extremely difficult to understand.

As ever, Appa had a simple and practical reason for his actions. In his childhood, meals were for sustenance and not for pleasure. You ate what was placed in front of you and were thankful for it. There were many going hungry around you. The woman—mother or aunt—in charge of the kitchen decided the meal and the portion, which was always meagre due to the large number of mouths to feed. And obviously there wasn't any variety. It was unheard of, for parents to ask their child what they wanted to eat or for a child to demand a particular dish. These were joint families with a limited budget and it just wasn't feasible.

Imagine placing the current generation of kids in this scenario. It would teach them a thing or two about wanting and wasting.

Anyway, after a while, when he could afford it, Appa starting eating a variety of things, wanting to sample everything that he couldn't in his childhood. I can imagine it even without having suffered a deprived childhood; I sometimes go crazy when it comes to food and it's just not me—I have seen the best of human beings turn into animals when hungry. I believe there is even an urban slang for it: being 'hangry'.

Well, as everyone knows, Appa is different. He is constantly growing and in a few years, he had had enough of the variety and the excess. Old tastes took centre stage again.

Variety can become confusing. In your haste to taste everything, you often miss out on enjoying what you truly like. By the time you have decided what you actually want, you are full. Or you are full before you have tasted everything and are left wondering whether the rest of it is better than what you have already had. Your taste buds grow jaded with the assault of flavours in that one meal and often give up. So actually sticking to one dish at every meal ensures that you enjoy every element that dish has to offer. Your stomach and your taste buds are not

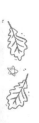

overwhelmed. You can gauge what you have eaten, how much you have eaten, and whether it was good for you (especially in these times, when counting calories is uppermost in everyone's mind). There is an innate satisfaction in the whole process.

I was quite young at that point and was still enamoured by the newness of things and the urge to try everything, so had a hard time understanding him. But of late, I have realized that Appa's philosophy towards food can be applied to life itself.

Variety has become almost a curse in the modern world. Just try ordering a normal coffee in a coffee shop. We are involuntarily teaching our kids that there is something better around every corner and in that process, they forget to appreciate the present. Instead, we should be telling them, make a choice and stick to it. Understand the value of what you possess. Life will always throw more at you. Know what to pick and what will make you happy in the long run. Be it food, family, love, career or even cranky cooks!

On a more practical note, I hope to incorporate health and simple cooking into my sons' mealtimes. What you eat when you are young defines your taste for a lifetime. (This is based on scientific research, mind you.) And that power is in my hands now as a mother. It is tough as hell, when pizzas, fried chicken and tons of addictive sugary foods compete for your children's attention, but I try my best to make them appreciate and understand the soul of food, rather than its fleeting pleasures.

Radio Ga Ga

If you grew up in the 1980s in India, radio would have been a huge part of your life. Cassette players and LPs were restricted to the affluent households. Television was yet to make inroads. The kids would hear it in the background while the mother moved around the kitchen, making breakfast and packing lunch. Old melodies would play on it while they got ready for school in the morning. It would play in the autos, cars and even cycle-rickshaws as they travelled to and from school. It was the background music in the evenings as they went for tuitions or to the playground. From news to sports commentary, film music to classical, everything was covered. If you were born in the seventies or early eighties, you are lucky to have been able to experience the best of the previous generation as well as the newer technological advances, from radio to cassette players to Walkmans, CD players and iPods, streaming and more.

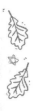

The radio influenced tastes in music and what started out as favourites then continue to dominate the current playlist for most people. Radio, I think, was instrumental in promoting film music and, happily, it is still around. Piped through speakers in malls, heard in cars during traffic jams, on phones, in teashops. From the singular All India Radio, it's now a bevy of stations broadcasting everything from regional music to talk shows.

I grew up never listening to the radio because my mother never listened to it. We had a huge tape recorder that was given pride of place next to the puja space in the living room. We weren't allowed to touch it. Amma would play the 'Vishnu Suprabhatham' every morning. It was the background score to my waking up and getting ready for school. The gadget would then go silent till the evening when bhajans or the 'Vishnu Sahasranamam' would play. I would walk in from my dance or tennis lessons, shower and sit down to do my homework, and it would be playing throughout. When we were young, Amma would teach us how to write with the help of a blackboard. The bhajans are the musical score for that memory.

Our car didn't have any cassette decks installed and the radio was never played when we travelled in it. Strange as it may sound, I had no idea what a radio was until much later in life.

I was learning the veena during my school days and was once invited to play at the All India Radio station in Madras. I had no idea what the place was about. I got there and was ushered into a small recording studio. When I finished playing, I asked my teacher when I could listen to it. She told me it would play on the radio at a particular time the next day. I told her I didn't have a radio at home. She stared at me and asked me to repeat what I had just said. I said again, I don't have a radio at home. Finally, looking extremely puzzled, she asked me to tell my mother what she had said and left it at that. I came home and repeated the instruction to my mother, who didn't bat an eyelid and said okay. I asked her if we had a radio and she pointed to the huge tape recorder I wasn't allowed to touch. 'That has a radio too.'

I asked her how it was operated and the next day, she showed me the buttons and dials that we fiddled with until the veena recital came on. The students' names were announced and the strains of the veena came through. Everyone gathered around to hear it, family and staff. At the end there was a round of applause from everyone, though I now realize that most of them were unlikely to have enjoyed it very much, compared to the peppy film songs they were used to hearing. All I was thinking of at that point was how I could learn to operate the radio. I tried the next morning, but there were too many buttons and dials. Disappointed, I decided it was a stupid gadget.

A few years later, Amma started practising yoga. She would bring the yoga mat to the living room early in the evening and do her asanas while music played lightly in the background. Oddly, she played Abba and the Beatles. Some days it was Roxette. Weekends also saw the tape recorder spewing out these seventies staples. I grew up listening to them and became strangely attached to the music. '*Hey Jude*' is a favourite track to this day. I also have a faint memory of the radio in my friend's house. She had a cook from Chettinad who used to play it in the kitchen. Their dining table was also in the kitchen and when we sat down to eat, the radio would be a lively accompaniment.

Ironically, film songs didn't enter my life until much later, not until I had reached my teens. Not even my father's movie scores. My mother had very different ideas about bringing us up (many of my childhood friends would use the word 'weird'). I can barely remember watching movies or even television when I was young. There were three TVs at home. A large Dyanora in my father's room, one in my parent's bedroom, and a smaller one in the living room for those working in the house to watch during their free time. I was only allowed to watch specific programmes and nothing during the week. Tamil films based on mythology or 'clean' black-and-white comedies. English classics like *The Sound of Music* or *My Fair Lady* were staples. They still remain

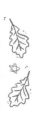

my favourites. As I grew up and listened to more film music, I became a big A.R. Rahman fan. He was a sensation then, and went on to win an Oscar, making us very proud.

I married a man who grew up listening only to the radio. Television was a luxury his family couldn't afford for a long time. The radio was also my mother-in-law's companion when the children were at school and her husband at work. It made her tedious day seem a little less so. Dhanush was an ardent fan of Illayaraja sir's music. He knew every song, every lyric and every background score that the maestro had created. Whenever he asked me whether I had heard a particular song, I would shake my head in embarrassment. He was shocked that despite being a part of the film community, I hadn't heard so many of the legend's compositions. I told him I knew Illayaraja sir and referred to him as 'uncle' but had not heard much of his music. I had spent so many lovely Navaratri evenings at his place and even accompanied Appa for music sittings. His son and I would play in the room while he was busy creating hit songs.

Dhanush was very amused and urged me to listen better. That was when I discovered Illayaraja sir's music and fell in love with it. One of my favourite songs is 'Panivizhum Malarvanam' (from the movie *Ninaivellam Nithya*). Dhanush also reintroduced me to the radio and we soon became inseparable. It accompanies me on the morning school commute, at the gym, and when I am stuck in endless traffic.

I also discovered a renewed interest in Tamil film music and, thankfully, can now hold my own in a conversation with my husband on that subject.

Childhood Friends

You don't need to be a celebrity child to know the dangers of having the wrong friends or the pleasures of a good one. As kids, my mother surrounded my sister and me with people she trusted, so that nobody could take advantage of us. It may seem weird to a normal person, but think back—didn't your parents censor your budding friendships, making sure the kids you spent time with had 'respectable' parents or were well behaved? My mother did the same, with a little extra focus. And thanks to her, my childhood friends have come to define my idea of friendship.

My sister is the one who collects friends wherever she goes; I am an extreme introvert, to the point of coming off as a snob. I am comfortable being alone and can never initiate a conversation or, for that matter, continue one with a stranger. That doesn't mean I don't have friends, I have had a number of them and they run the entire spectrum. I can't name most them, of course, but I am sure many of you can relate to these descriptions. I hope my friends and acquaintances aren't mortified by my metaphors, but this is how I've often categorized them in my head.

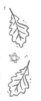

Water on a lotus leaf—Touch and go without leaving any memories.

Cats and dogs—Always fighting but connected by a strange bond and get along irrespective of traditional enmity.

Flower and butterfly—The flower gives, the butterfly takes and flies away.

The ocean—Vast, deep and forever, unconditional.

The project friendships—Last as long as the project, the employment together, the holiday together, etc.

The social friendship—Friends who meet only at social gatherings.

As I mentioned earlier, Amma was wary of anyone who wanted to become friends with us. She constantly drilled the need for caution into our heads and surrounded us with people she approved of so that we did not feel the need to make friends outside. Every Saturday, a group of trusted friends and cousins were invited home. She planned activities, games, story-telling, puzzles and much more that filled our days. Picnics to beaches, parks and temples were also planned. We ate, napped, played and fought together, almost twenty kids of different ages. It was the highlight of our week. If the parents planned anything for the evening, it would include us too. As the evenings stretched into the night, we were all bundled into a room and the TV was switched on. Indiana Jones was a favourite. Back-to-back Indiana Jones movies with a constant supply of snacks from the kitchen is one of my cherished childhood memories.

As we grew older, the group reduced considerably in size. Some became too old for our childish games, most made friends at school or in their neighbourhoods and wanted to spend more time with them. My sister and I also grew up and Amma began to trust us to choose our friends wisely. But that time spent together stayed with us. A few of us still meet once in a while, trying to relive those carefree days. Two of those childhood friends have become my soul sisters (if I can be excused such a corny term). Poornima and Sriya are my 3 a.m. buddies, my pillars of support and lifesavers. They don't care if I let weeks go by without calling or meeting. They know, just as well as I do, that we can catch up where we left off in a second. They know me inside out.

When we were children, I thought I shared a weird telepathic bond with Poornima. We would think of the same things at the same time and react to things in the exact same manner. It was eerie. It happens even now. We are so much in sync, it's scary. I remember we used to force our mothers to dress us up in similar clothes.

Poornima is part of the illustrious Naidu Hall family and went on to do great things. Sriya, on the other hand, was a real tomboy, fearless and outgoing. She would constantly be on the field playing football or talking nonstop about cricket. (Her father is the former Indian cricketer Bharat Reddy.) Ironically, Poorni and I were the ones who played dress-up but it was Sriya who grew up to become the fashionista. Both of them are Telugu and can be blamed for my love of spicy pickles and fiery Andhra food. Poornima also has the distinction of being the only friend in whose house I was allowed to spend a night!

The two of them filled my life and it never even crossed my mind to glance outside this close-knit circle when it came to friendships. Poornima's father used to race as a hobby and she learnt how to drive very early on. They had a fancy open-top car and her father allowed her to take it on short drives. When she first offered to take us with her, everyone agreed, except Amma. She was mortified. No way was she going to allow me a ride in an open-top car, through the city, driven by a young girl. One evening, when Poornima came visiting with the car, Amma wasn't at home. In an unusually impulsive move, I got in and we went for a spin. That drive along the Marina, with the wind blowing in my hair and the stolen freedom is one of my favourite memories.

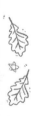

I had never, until then, travelled in an open vehicle on a public road. The journey Appa started as a bus conductor and which resulted in him becoming a superstar ensured that I could never travel in a bus myself. The irony!

The first drive was the sweetest and the scariest. After that I would go to her place and ask her to take me for a round as many times as I could get away with it, and she took me whenever she could. After her father passed away, she sold the car and did not drive for a very long time.

I had to learn to drive rather sneakily. It was pretty late in life. One of our trusted drivers, who had been with us for years, taught me on the sly in a compact little Hyundai Santro, which had just been launched then. This used to happen on the way back from my dance classes. It was my friend's comfort with cars that spurred me to learn.

As adults too, my best friends have become my pride and joy. Sriya started out as a hugely popular VJ and went on to make her mark in movies. Her performance in *Thimuru* and *Kanchivaram* were critically acclaimed, her rustic characters in those films miles apart from the stylish young woman that she is. Ironically Sriya is now the homebody and Poornima went on to win a National award for costume design for the period drama *Paradesi* after she had married and settled down with a child. Not only did my friends enrich my childhood, they inspire me to do better even now.

My early childhood, as I have said before, was spent in Bangalore, with my grandparents. We lived in an apartment block that had two flats on each floor. Opposite our house lived a boy called Shankar and below us, on the first floor, were two children, Pallavi and Pranay. Shankar is a year younger to me, Pranay is almost a year older. Pallavi and my sister are the same age. These were my first friends. The usual games brought us together—robber and police, lock and key, and an invented game called pole to pole. There were a large number of pillars in the car park of the apartment and we numbered them. The goal of the game was to touch the pillar that the catcher called out the number of, without being caught. There were other kids in the neighbouring buildings, but they weren't allowed to get out of their compound and we weren't allowed to leave ours, so it was just the four of us. I left Bangalore when I was around nine, but the friendship endured. We lost touch with Shankar when he moved away but Pranay and I, who were the nearest in age, became the closest. I would call him when I was low, for advice, for reassurance, and he always responded in the most non-judgemental fashion. As a matter of fact, I recommend a close friend of the opposite gender for everyone. Makes relationships so much easier to understand!

Appa was initially very wary, in his own traditional, orthodox way. He would not allow Pranay to call after 6 p.m. or let us meet without a chaperone once I entered my teens, which was rather funny because our relationship was strictly platonic. Amma, in her usual all-knowing motherly way, knew there was nothing to be worried about and usually left us to our devices. I think she realized that in a home full of women, I needed a male friend to navigate the world.

When I decided to get married, Pranay was one of the first to know. He was close enough to tell me I was crazy to marry at such a young age, only to immediately change his mind when he met Dhanush. Pranay knew me well enough to realize Dhanush was perfect for me. He came for the wedding and was there from start to finish, alongside my own family. Appa now looks at him with affection, no doubt wondering why he had made such a fuss when we were younger.

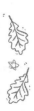

Over the years, I must admit there have been times when I blamed Amma for my reserved nature. Did her words of caution keep me from trusting people or being friendly? But then, my sister, who was brought up in the same atmosphere, makes friends everywhere she goes and from all walks of life. Whereas I feel like there is a line I cannot cross until I know the person really well. I am more content with the few real friends I have, than a large number of acquaintances, though I do envy extroverts and their ease with people. Then, one day, it struck me: it was nature, not nurture. Appa is also reserved and I remember only a few people who are regulars at home and with whom my father chats freely. I now relate to that feeling of security that only a few people can bring. For me it is my childhood friends, for Appa it is people who stood by him when he left Bangalore, the ones with whom he shared his first smoke and his first drink, those who sold their belongings to help him realize his dreams and, of course, a select few from the film industry who were there for him while he grew as an actor.

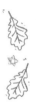

Pet Peeves

Dogs, cats, birds, fish, rabbits and even snakes, pets are an integral part of many people's lives. I know some who are more attached to their pets than to the humans around them. I don't get it. I am petrified of animals. I have never been bitten or chased or even seen any animal being mean to humans, but the fear is real. Something so deep that the only way I can be around dogs, which most of my friends have, is when they are held on a leash, at a distance. I do appreciate them, but usually with ten feet of space and a wall or a gate between us. Maybe it's genetic: I have a cousin who is so scared of cats that she gets a fever after every encounter. My own phobia is such that I call ahead when visiting homes with pets so that they can be kept away from me. When going to places where I am not sure about their presence, I wait outside the gate until I can confirm with the watchman or anyone around. I do feel bad for the dogs and cats that have been locked into a room just because I am around, but it's either that or a cardiac arrest for me.

When I was around eleven or twelve, my grandparents would take me with them when visiting an uncle who lived in Singapore. It was very exciting; he had a lovely house with a beautiful backyard with lots of birds, which I was fine with, because birds kept their distance. There was a dog too. The first time I saw him, I ran for my life. The second time I saw him, I did the same. After it had happened a couple of times more, they realized my fear was real and kept the dog in the backyard until I left on the sightseeing jaunt for the day with my grandparents. One day, the dog was on its daily walk and I was enjoying myself in the backyard, which I had all to myself, when I happened to look into the neighbour's yard. It had a beautiful garden, with flowers in bloom and a fountain in the corner. There was a huge cage at the end of the garden. It was empty, except for a large rock in one corner. My uncle had just walked out into the yard and I asked him what animal usually occupied the cage. He laughed and asked me to look carefully. What I had thought was a rock, was a fat, eight-foot python snoozing in the sun. I literally jumped onto my uncle, and he held me for a moment as I processed the craziness! The holiday went for a toss. I kept imagining the owner leaving the cage open and the python that had been on a diet of birds and rats, craving for something more substantial. Like the little girl who had come to visit next door.

Over the years, I visited my uncle a couple more times and the python was always there in the neighbour's house. Then, on one visit, I came to know that it had died and the owner was heartbroken. Apparently he continued to mourn the snake for years after that. I could only think that if he could feel that kind of love for a snake that just ate and lay in the sun, people with dogs must be devastated to lose them, they offer such unconditional love. One more reason to stay away from pets, I thought. I couldn't handle the heartbreak.

As I said earlier, the problem must be genetic because my grandmother wasn't too fond of dogs either, nor was my mother. So I never had one growing up, either in Bangalore or later, in Madras. The only animals that I saw were the cats that roamed around outside the house, looking for scraps. They seemed more afraid of me than I was of them. When my sister and I were in our teens, she made friends with a bunch of schoolmates who had dogs at home. After every visit, she would come home and rave about the special bond that the pets had with the kids in the house. She would go on and on about how we had missed out on that whole experience in our childhood. About how much love they had to offer and how beautiful it was. Appa loves dogs too, and she found an ally in her quest. Together they managed to convince Amma and we brought home our first pet. His name was Tiger Rajinikanth.

Tiger was the sweetest Dalmatian and the first pet I ever touched. Since he was a puppy when he came, I didn't feel threatened, though I kept my distance. And how could one not get caught up in the excitement of having a new baby at home, feeding, playing, scratching and chewing things all over the place. I remember we were so enamoured by him, we used to check on him even in the middle of the night to see if he was fine. He was so friendly that even I would feed him sometimes and let him follow me around. Appa and my sister were ecstatic and it was nice seeing them so happy.

Tiger grew up pretty fast and was a very lively dog, but in his own intelligent doggy way, he understood my fears. He would play rough with everyone else, jumping on them and demanding to be petted. With me he would just come close, wag his tail, sniff around a bit and leave, having made sure that I noticed his acknowledgement of me. Tiger was the only pet I was comfortable with. And who could resist his doggy smile?

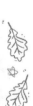

Though it was my sister and father who insisted on bringing home a dog, it was Amma who eventually became closest to him. Appa had a busy schedule and my sister had school, so inevitably he ended up spending most of his time with Amma. She was a typical homemaker, whose life revolved around the three of us and the house. Once a pet arrived, she became even more so. She did not like travelling much and now she had a perfect excuse. She had to stay home and take care of the dog. Tiger followed her around everywhere and even mimicked her food habits. He was a vegetarian dog who loved paneer and curd rice! We used to tell her that dogs needed their non-vegetarian protein and feeding him only vegetarian food was unfair, but she wouldn't listen, so Appa used to slip him some meat once in a while without her knowledge and Tiger loved it. It was only after many years that Amma allowed dog food into the house.

Once, we had to leave for an extended stretch and it was unavoidable. Appa had a rare break and we decided to go on a holiday to Singapore. After a lot of thought, a caretaker was arranged for Tiger and we left. Amma used to call him every day to make sure Tiger was all right and he told her each time that her dog was fine. When we came back, Tiger was strangely subdued. I felt he looked sad. Amma called the doctor, who said he was physically perfect. But we were not convinced, so we called the caretaker, who said nothing had happened. But as he was speaking to Amma, Tiger lunged at him and bit his hand. It was the first time he had ever behaved aggressively. Amma was stunned and shouted at him. The caretaker was taken immediately to a hospital and both Amma and Tiger went into a sulk. She refused to eat and so did he.

That evening, the night watchman who had been with us for years spoke to my mother. I heard her cry out and then run and hug Tiger. The caretaker had fooled us all. He had treated Tiger badly a couple of times, even beating him. Tiger had not retaliated until we were back and he knew he was safe. It was almost as though he had waited for us to come back before giving the guy what he deserved. The man was given a dressing-down and fired, but the damage was done. Tiger had become wary of strangers.

In a household where people come and go regularly, like ours, it became torturous for him and for us. He was extremely temperamental and stressed and it came to a point where he would randomly attack people. Finally, the doctor we always took him to, told us that he would foster him so that he could spend the rest of his days away from the triggers that made him paranoid. I did not realize how much a part of the family he had become until he left. It was hard on all of us, especially Amma. We would go to visit him and come back feeling even more dejected than before. It just didn't feel right. A week later, nobody could take it anymore. A huge fenced lawn was prepared for him and he was brought back home. He lived for thirteen years and though he spent most of his time in that fenced portion, he was at least close to us and he seemed happy to be away from strangers. In scarring a dog, the caretaker had scarred an entire family.

Tiger had mated once and we had got one pup out of the litter. (Apparently, that's the norm. The male's family gets one pup and the female's family keeps the rest.) The pup was sent to our farmhouse in the outskirts of the city and so there was always one descendant of Tiger there. Whenever there was a new litter, the caretaker at the farm would bring the one we were keeping to the house. Amma would name the puppy and it would return to the farm where they all lived happily. This went on for a while. One day, the caretaker came home with a tiny little thing that my mother named Nanda. Just then, he got the news that someone in his family was sick and he had to leave immediately. He said he would come back for the pup after two days. Nanda never left.

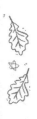

Nanda, just like Tiger, knew my limits. He knew I loved him, I knew he adored me too, but there was no petting. He soon became my mother's shadow. After my sister and I got married and left home, he was left alone with my mother. He was there when I had my two babies and he was there when my grandfather passed away. But all good things have to come to an end and after thirteen years of giving us unconditional love, he passed away. Amma swore then, never to have another dog in the house. She had gone through the trauma of losing one, twice over, and was sure that she couldn't do it again.

Dogs are like saints in a way. Teaching us life lessons while asking only for affection in return. Love them and they love you back tenfold. They slowly become part of your life and give it a new meaning. It is unfortunate that my fear of them has stopped me from experiencing the completeness of such a lovely relationship. My husband, on the other hand, grew up with dogs and loves them. Not long after we met, I gifted him a Labrador puppy that was hell on paws, a tiny boy that stole my heart. But fate had other plans. The puppy came down with an infection and passed away. It had a huge impact on me. I decided it was a sign that dogs and I were not meant to be. Our lives are already so full of relationships that come with expectations. Some of these relationships are not a matter of choice, others we choose, some out of love and some out of need. A relationship with a dog is different. I do not know whether I can do full justice to its unconditional love. And this voluntary attachment that has such a short life makes me uncomfortable.

As a mother I would love for my children to have a pet. It is a rite of passage that makes people more empathetic. Dhanush also feels it is a bond that children should experience and I am being selfish in letting my fears get in the way. The mother in me says yes, the little girl in me screams no, and the homemaker in me reminds me of my white sofas and wooden flooring. Once I came close to asking them who they wanted in the house—a puppy or me? The sentence didn't make it out of my mouth because I was pretty sure they would have settled for the dog. But the best-laid plans have a tendency to go awry, and as you read this, I may or may not have caved in and acquired another four-legged fountain of love in my life.

Decoding My Day

Night is upon me and I sit swaddled in the shadows of the room, trying to decode my day. Rewinding to the moment I opened my eyes at the break of dawn. Lying there and trying to squeeze out a few extra minutes under the covers. There has never been a day when I didn't want to snooze for a little more time. I think about the day ahead and hope it is like our weather, which is almost always predictable—blue skies and sunshine. But life has shown me that I can never know what is in store for me. I go through the routine, some things done out of habit, some out of love, and some that I just want to get through. The kids packed off to school, my better half off to work and my workout out of the way, household duties beckon. The cook is given the menu for the day, instructions are handed out for tidying up and I am out of the door. There are schedules to plan, deadlines to meet. Inefficiency to blow my top at and consistency to greet enthusiastically. By midday, I crave a break and head to my mother's place—to have lunch and to be bullied to eat more. Amma is serving us food and Appa is in a fun mood. Good food and great conversation. A bit of teasing, a few old memories and, of course, gossip galore.

I look out of the window, happy with my lot, and everything fades into the background as I see her pottering about. A tiny old lady, raking leaves under the mango tree. She is smiling softly,

84

the lines deep and etched into her wrinkled face. Like someone took the woman I remembered and crumpled her in the palm of their hands. But she is content, lines and all. She has seen me crawling around on all fours, sent me off to school. She has seen me getting married and seen my children crawl and then play around. I am greedy; I want her to go through the same cycle with them.

I have never seen her idle, she is always working at something or the other, never frowning. I know for certain that her heart has never held anything bitter or false. She does not have any gold or silver on her, just a head covered in grey. She looks so fragile and small, it evokes a feeling so deep, so raw. A feeling I seldom experience, even for my near and dear ones. She looks up, notices me and smiles. It tells a story of all that has gone past her, of all the love and care that she has to offer. A smile that is brighter than a Chennai afternoon in summer. A smile that warms the heart. There are no words exchanged. She goes on with her work and I get on with my day. It's late, the children are snug in bed and I am in my room swaddled in the shadows, decoding my day. I sit still for a while and realize, the best part of my day was that tender smile.

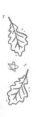

a Fan

His name was Karthik.

He was part of a Rajinikanth fan club. Appa has five main fan clubs and numerous smaller ones across the world. So what does a fan club do? Apart from the usual first day, first show, first row madness, they do a lot of community work. Like any other club, it's a gathering of people who share similar interests—and in this case, it's Rajinikanth the actor.

It is just before a movie releases that a fan club truly comes into its own. Festivities are organized; social service activities such as blood donation drives, health awareness drives, etc., are conducted. This is something that sets apart fan clubs in Tamil Nadu from others around the world. The day before the release, they go around the city to check on the humungous hoardings and cut-outs, make sure their members have their T-shirts (bought from their own pooled resources) and put the festoons and arrangements in place for the aarti and the milk bathing of the cut-outs. Some spend the night in a theatre, to make sure they get the first tickets. It is exciting, festive and fun! I do not find it strange at all, mostly because I grew up with it. A movie release has always been an occasion to be enjoyed.

I remember Karthik from such an occasion. He had joined the fan club in 1978 and soon become an integral part of it. When I was around ten, he came home with five boys from the main fan clubs and that was the first time I saw him. Amma treated them like they were her children and they reciprocated the affection. He was tall and dark, with light eyes and a demeanour that made him stand out from the rest. He looked intimidating, but as we got to know him, I realized he was a gentle soul.

The boys would visit not just during movie release time, but also otherwise, spending time at Appa's office, sometimes as often as twice in a month. It was not necessary for Appa to be around. They would turn up and help out with anything that was happening at that point. If it was lunch time, Amma would invite them to eat with the office staff. The happy part of it was that they respected our privacy. Never did we feel that they crossed a line into our space. They loved to spend some time around the place where Appa lived, and that was all. It was unconditional love for my father with no expectations in return. At public functions, they would volunteer as bodyguards, forming a protective cordon around my sister, mother and me, keeping us safe when the crowds got too close. There were times when the crowds would get physically intimidating, even hurting these boys with their pushing and shoving, but they protected us. My sister and I became the siblings they never had, and even if they had siblings, I doubt they would have taken care of them the way they took care of us. None of them would accept anything in return. We tried offering money, clothes and other things, but they felt insulted. As far as they were concerned, we were family and they were doing it out of love.

Karthik was the special one. Back then, Appa would meet his fans in the morning before heading for the day's shoot and Karthik would be there most of the time, helping control the crowd if there were too many, or making people stand in an orderly line for pictures. He would be having a cup of coffee, supplied from Amma's ever bountiful kitchen, and I would be getting ready for school or to study. He would give me an encouraging nod before heading out. Karthik would be the one standing next to me when we watched Appa's films at a theatre or went out. He often remarked on how much I resembled Appa. (Which must have contributed in some way to the affection he had for me.)

Karthik got a steady job working at the Slum Clearance Board and he was a loving son to his family. First appearances aside (he could come across as coarse and arrogant), he was unfailingly warm and responsible. He soon got married to a sweet girl called Nirmala. After the wedding ceremony, they came to meet Appa. When he asked them if they had gone to a temple to get blessings after the ceremony, he replied, 'That's why I have come here.'

Time went by and Karthik had three daughters, he was a doting father and a good husband, but his love for Appa came first. His family understood that, even embraced it. He visited often and was always at the forefront of the movie release festivities. There was just one thing that he did not do for us. Karthik used to drink occasionally, but he had the bad habit of drinking and then driving his bike home. He was not an alcoholic, just enjoyed his drink once in a while. He was not the type who would get drunk and create a ruckus, in public or at home, so people usually did not stop him from driving. His wife was concerned, but he did not listen to her. Amma tried, but he wouldn't listen to her either.

In 1995, *Muthu* was released and we all got back from the first show, ecstatic at the response. Appa never comes to a theatre, he waits at home and listens to our discussions on how the audience responded. We were sure the film was a winner. The boys (by now grown men) were also present and they filled the backyard, happiness and pride on their faces. It was like Appa had not let them down, they could still hold their heads high as members of his fan club.

Amma arranged for lunch and everyone dug in. Karthik ate, silent as usual, but beaming with joy. He finished and came up to me to say something, a sheen of happy tears in his eyes, then hesitated and turned away. I was distracted by something at that moment and forgot about it. I wish I had not. In a while, they all left, Karthik looking extremely happy and animated. It was a common effect after watching a Rajini movie. I have seen the magic too many times to count. I waved goodbye. Little did I know it would be the last time I was seeing my father's favourite fan.

That evening, one of the office staff came running to my mother and whispered something to her. Amma turned a horrible shade of grey, then ran to Appa's room, and I followed her, knowing something really bad had happened. Karthik had gone to a local bar after leaving our house. He had a couple more drinks than usual and as he was driving his bike back home, it skidded on some loose soil and he fell. He passed away on the spot.

A pall of gloom fell over the house. It was too much for me to take. After a few hours of disbelief, all I could do was rant. It was not fair! Why would god do something like that? Appa mourned in silence.

I kept thinking over the events of the day, the number of times we had warned him. Should we have been more forceful? Why did his friends let him drive when they knew he had drunk more than usual? He was so sensible about everything else in his life, why not this? Eventually I had to stop and accept the reality of it. Appa had lost a dear fan, Amma a foster son and my sister and I, our guardian angel. God takes away good people too soon, their part in the world much shorter but sweeter.

It took us a long time to get over Karthik's senseless death. He was more than a fan, he was family.

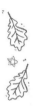

Madras, Movies and the Maestro

Madras, as it was called then and is still called in the innermost musings of my mind, was once the hub of regional movies in the south. Telugu, Malayalam, Kannada and Tamil movies were all shot and processed in Madras. The city had numerous film studios and flourishing production houses catering to all the southern languages. The bigger hotels had celebrities walking in and out. The busy stars who had families moved to the city as they would be shooting here almost all year round. Shooting in faraway locations was rare; films were mostly shot on sets in film studios. Their children went to school in Madras and I can count a number of friends that I grew up with whose parents were from the Telugu and Kannada film industries. You can see proof of this in most of the star kids of the Telugu and Malayalam industries; they all speak extremely good Tamil.

Since most of the shoots in those days took place indoors, there was no concept of vanity vans, only makeup and changing rooms. Appa therefore finds it very odd to wait in vanity vans and often pulls up a chair and sits outside, next to where the shoot is happening. The fact that this also keeps him up to date on all aspects of shooting, he can see how the other actors are faring and what's actually happening in the movie, is secondary. The primary result of this is that there is camaraderie on the set, a feeling that everyone is involved, and it shows when the final product is screened.

This camaraderie was apparent in the big studios of the day: AVM, Vijaya Vauhini, Prasad, Sathya, Mohini and many more. If you were to walk in on any working day, there would be a Rajkumar shoot happening at one end, an NTR shoot at the other, and an MGR shoot in between. When the different crews broke for lunch, they would all gather together and eat, beyond language, star power and other barriers. This continued with Appa's generation. They shared a special rapport that went beyond movies. Fans who waited outside the studios to see their favourite star would get a glimpse of others stars too. However clichéd it may sound, they were one big family working under the same roof.

One thing that has changed dramatically over the years is the role of the producer. Appa tells me that in those days, the producer would be on set the entire time. He was usually very well informed when it came to technicalities such as camerawork, as well as the creative aspects of movie-making. He would provide inputs, put out the minor flare-ups that are a normal part of film-making and also help the team overcome any problems they had. These producers were capable men who knew what they were doing and how to get their money's worth.

Among them were stalwarts who were known for their reliability and expertise. Except for the more recent films, Appa has never signed a contract or an agreement. A word was enough. A handshake was as binding as a tightly written, signed and witnessed agreement.

There was one particular producer whose story thrilled me every time Appa spoke about it.

Let's call him Producer T. His banner was so well respected, it was considered an honour to be booked under it. He once hired a well-known director from another language industry to helm one of his movies in Tamil. The shoot took place in one of his studios in Madras. The script called for a large cast and the production budget was huge. Producer T had a lot of money at stake. He would come every day and stay till pack-up, antsy and nervous. Others from the film fraternity who were shooting at the same studio would come around to pay their respects during the breaks and wish him luck. This went on for a few days.

A certain sequence for the film required a massive, and expensive, set and its fabrication was in progress. The producer called one of the assistant directors and asked him to narrate the scene that was to be shot on this set. He then called the art director and recommended a few changes. The art director was impressed but mentioned that it would cost a lot more. 'I think the scene deserves it, do whatever it takes,' was the response he got. The entire team was shocked. Budgets running out of hand usually made producers angry, but here was Producer T, opting to spend more. The incident endeared him to everyone on the set and the shoot proceeded smoothly. Everyone except the director. He wasn't very happy having the producer on set all day, especially a producer who recommended changes that the art director carried out without question. He wasn't used to the style of working in Madras and would complain constantly: 'The producer's job is to put money into the film and await the results. His job is not to interfere. Besides, what does a producer know about making movies?'

Those who knew the producer tried to dissuade him from this stance. They told him about the expertise and experience Producer T had, but their words fell on deaf ears and it all came to a head one day.

The shoot was in progress and Producer T was sitting in a corner with the accountant, going over the expenses. His ears listened to the accountant's explanations but his eyes were on the shoot. Something struck him as odd and he beckoned to the assistant director and asked him to narrate the scene. Producer T was silent for a while and then suggested some changes. He asked the assistant director to run these by the director and then make the changes. The guy was hesitant. Making changes to a set while it was being constructed was one thing, asking for a change during the shoot was another thing altogether. How would an already antagonized director react to this? He was stuck between the devil and the deep sea. He couldn't refuse the producer who was financing the film and at the same time he couldn't afford to annoy his direct boss, the director. His career depended on these people. He stood there undecided and the expression on his face must have been telling, because Producer T told him to relax and went over to the director himself.

The director was speaking to the heroine of the film. She was a stunner, as were most actresses of that era. As Producer T came up, he realized the director was not discussing the scene or the movie, but generally chatting her up, and she was too well behaved to ignore him. He went up to them and laid out his apprehensions about the scene. He was very straightforward about it and didn't mince his words. The entire set froze. This was the first time the producer had approached the director, asking for changes to be made. They had all heard the director complain about the producer's interference and wondered what was going to happen next.

The director got up from his chair to face Producer T, looked him in the eye and said, 'What do you know about film-making, sir?'

There were audible gasps from those around them.

Producer T didn't bat an eyelid.

'I am a film-maker. I know what I need to do and how a shot needs to be taken and how my film should look. You are just the producer who puts in the money for creative people like me to make films to entertain audiences. You are only supposed to do that. I will not accept anyone coming to my set and instructing me on how I should be making my film. I will give you the respect that a producer requires, but nothing more. Please step aside, sir. You have no understanding of how a film is made. You might have the knowledge of how to sell it, but not of how to create it. I am the creator here. Do you understand me?'

Everyone present there was aghast. The senior members of the unit shook their heads and muttered at the director's impunity. Some of the youngsters, new to the field, thought the director was gutsy to have spoken up against the system. Most just waited to see what would happen next.

Producer T smiled and walked away. Those who were waiting for fireworks were disappointed. The director was ecstatic that he'd had the last say, that too in front of the fetching heroine. Pack-up was announced.

The next day, everyone arrived early to see what would happen. Would the producer appear? How would the director react? The tension was intense. The director walked in and started giving instructions for the day's shoot. Work started slowly, building up tempo by mid-morning. The actors arrived and were ushered into the makeup rooms. The costume department was on its toes, getting the large cast ready for the scene. The catering department had started serving hot breakfast and the bustle soon matched that of a busy, productive set. Yet, at the back of everyone's mind, the same thought ran. The man who usually came to the set before everyone else was missing today. Producer T.

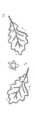

After the first half of the day was done, that thought found its voice. Would the missing producer withdraw from the film? Was he sick? Had he given up so easily? What did his absence mean? The director's curiosity couldn't be contained any longer, either. He asked the production manager, who ignored the question and walked away.

The next day, all the leading newspapers had a massive front-page advertisement announcing a new film under Producer T's banner. The artists were well known and the director was Producer T himself.

Later in the week, the unit came to know that the shoot had begun next door in the same studio. It created a storm of gossip unlike anything ever before. Forget the usual gossip about who was having a clandestine affair with whom, all talk turned to the two movies being shot simultaneously. One that had a huge budget and a new-age director, the other being directed by a producer and shrouded in secrecy.

The shoot lasted fifty days, and no outsider was allowed in during this time. Nothing was leaked out. The producer had not showed his face to anyone during the shoot, nor did he during the post-production stage. The only people who saw him were the crew of the film and they were loyal, not breathing a word. The entire industry was intrigued. Strange rumours flew about, including one that said he had hired a shadow director to direct the movie while he put his name on the masthead. This was put to rest after some of the members of the unit insisted that Producer T was calling the shots and was the sole captain of the ship. Another director bemoaned the waste of money just to prove a point and massage a producer's ego.

The big-budget film had been under production for six months and was still being shot. Producer T's film was ready for release in three months, during which time he did not visit the other set even once. From scripting to post-production, everything was done with a minimum of fuss but the end results were stunning. The movie released and was a super hit. Not only did it recover costs, it also made a very healthy profit for the producer.

A week after the release, when the film had been declared a runaway hit and there could be no doubts about its collection or the good reviews it had garnered, Producer T walked onto the young director's set.

When Producer T walked in, the aura of victory around him was unmistakable. He strode towards his usual corner, and someone brought him his chair. He sat and watched, just as he used to before. One by one, everyone went up to him during the break and spoke to him. The heroine came in from the makeup room and spotting the producer, ran up to him and offered her congratulations. The director ignored all this. He didn't have the courage to meet Producer T face to face.

Lunch break was called. Producer T got up from his chair and approached the director. The entire set waited, without leaving for lunch, to see the drama unfold. He got to where the director stood and looked into his eyes.

'Now can I make changes to the scene, son?' he asked.

The director could not reply.

Appa was shooting next-door that day and Producer T joined him for lunch, during the course of which he recounted the entire story.

The contentious scene was reshot and that film became a hit too. The scene that had caused all this trouble was talked about for its brilliance for a long time, both in the industry as well as among fans.

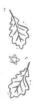

Once Upon a Scandal

Rumours, gossip, hook-ups, breakups. The film industry is known to supply fodder for innumerable stories, true or not. Whether one likes it or not, the curiosity surrounding the industry is such that people are always interested in hearing what is going on in their favourite celebrities' lives. Our lives are scrutinized, criticized and commented upon on a regular basis. In fact there is an entire industry that has grown around it. Most people in the limelight get used to it, some master the art of working around it and there are, of course, those geniuses who manage to stay out of it. Nobody goes around looking for gossip, but let's face it, one word here or there, and we get hooked. It's human nature. And I am sure this is true of every kind of space, not just the movies. The only difference is that when it comes to the movies, people think that because they have invited an onscreen character into their living rooms or spent time with them in the theatre, their personal life is fair game too.

I am no saint. It is always interesting to hear about who is dating or hooking up with whom, ego clashes on the set, cold wars among the stars, opportunistic friends, friends turned foes, foes turned BFFs and more. It's interesting because I am in the same industry and also because, let's face it, who can resist some juicy gossip once in a while.

But there is one story that goes beyond gossip for me. It's from an age when things were truly kept under wraps. No mobile phones to capture tender moments or scandalous proximity and instantly transmit them to the world. I remember the evenings when the uncles and aunties of the older generation would sit around after dinner and talk. I would be in a corner, drowsing, unnoticed but listening. And this story captured my imagination with its star-crossed lovers.

Once upon a time, in the golden era of Tamil cinema, there was a leading lady. She was young and talented. She was stunning to look at. She was everything a leading man could ask for.

He was a devoted family man with five children and a happy home. Respected for his talent and his principles.

They were offered a movie together, but she was hesitant. Her cronies whispered in her ears, 'You can't work with him, he is not one of us, he is not our friend.' The lady hated anyone telling her what to do. She was as spunky as she was beautiful. 'I was just mildly interested in the beginning, but now I will work with him. Do not tell me how to run my career. Besides, he is a decent family man, I have nothing to fear from him.'

The fates must have been laughing at her statement.

The shoot began and the leading man, who had not once looked at the bevy of beauties that surrounded him in the industry, who had stayed true to his wife through five children, fell head over heels in love with his leading lady.

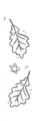

She was attached to an airline pilot and was envisioning a future with him, but her hero on reel became her bane in real life. She tried resisting, but he was besotted. He pursued her with a vengeance, refusing to give up even when she refused every advance. He became so obsessed with her that cracks began to appear in his family life. The heroine was alarmed and tried to cut off all ties with him, but he couldn't stop thinking, eating, sleeping and working with her in his heart. He was possessed by the thought of her, he believed that she was his true love, his soulmate.

The poor woman. He slowly broke down her barriers with his relentless pursuit. She was confused by the fact that ignoring him, insulting him, lashing out at him, pleading with him, rejecting him, only made him more persistent. He claimed to feel an extraordinary love for her, a bond that spanned lifetimes.

She gave in.

The wife, the wronged woman, who was confident of her husband's love, finally broke. Even when he was besotted with the other woman, she had thought that he would come back once the infatuation ran its course. She was lulled into a false sense of security because the other woman in question was not interested. But the equation had changed. A beautiful heroine had captured her husband's heart and he had captured her attention too.

Hell hath no fury like a woman scorned, and she proved it. He would come to the shoot with tears in his eyes. She spared nothing in her wrath. She had her children in her corner and would fight tooth and nail to get their father back.

It wreaked havoc in everyone's lives.

Particularly in our heroine's life. She said to the man, for whom she had given up her previous relationship, for whom she had braved the scandal that society was sure to throw at them, 'I can't bear to see you go through this, my love. I know you are fighting for me, but it's taking its toll on you, beyond what I expected.'

'As long as I have you by my side, I can take anything. As long as I know I will be with you in the end, I can live with anything now,' he replied.

'Even though it's hurting everyone around you and most of all—you?'

'I want you, I want to be with you, no matter what …'

She heard him out silently and left.

He tried to get in touch with her, but he couldn't. She had fallen off the radar. He went crazy. People still talk in whispers about the way he cried, wanting to hear her voice, how he ranted, wanting to catch a glimpse of her.

A few days later, he too disappeared. Everyone was frantic. His family needed him, there was a huge amount of money invested in him, which would be lost if he didn't turn up for work. As everyone ran from pillar to post trying to locate his whereabouts, his friend received a call.

'It's me. I cannot function without talking to her. I know she left because she couldn't bear to see my pain, but I can't bear life without her. I'll come back on one condition. She has to speak to me. Else I'll stay away. Live my entire life in hiding.'

The friend realized that people's livelihoods depended on the hero getting his heroine, so he convinced the lady and she relented. After all, she too was deeply in love.

She cried her heart out and called her love back. They believed it was the end of their travails, they believed they would never part again. They believed they belonged together. They were wrong.

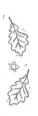

The wife refused to let go. She reached out to her family, his family, friends, colleagues. She reminded everyone of the marriage vows he had taken, to which they were witness. She paraded her children in front of them and demanded their rights. She threatened to end her life, along with her children's. Everyone sided with her; after all, it was a case of taking away a father from five children. So finally, society had its say. The hero bowed down to the pressure from all sides and decided that his one true love had to be sacrificed for the life of his children. Moreover, his lady love understood. She didn't stand a chance; she couldn't take him away from his children. They parted and he had to swear on his babies' heads that he would not pursue her.

She would have to live with the consolation that he loved her like no one else had, or would; that he would never love anyone else as much as he loved her.

I don't know how much of this story is fact and how much fiction, but sitting among those dazzling men and women who flamed across the screen, listening to their tales of love and lust, envy and redemption, I imagined a love written in the stars but not destined to last on earth.

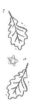

Perseverance

My first son was obsessed with Lego blocks, like many other kids of his age. We had once bought him an airplane set and he was playing with it at home. One wing of the plane just refused to stay in place. He tried everything, dismantling it, redoing it, trying it from various angles. Appa noticed his preoccupation and tried to distract him. It would work for a while but soon enough, the boy would get back to the wing. I was just thankful for the rare quiet time that I was getting (those with toddlers will surely understand) but Appa wanted to spend time with his grandson and kept luring him away. He finally gave up and the child went on until he managed to fit the wing on the plane, at which point we all rejoiced with him. The look on his face, of complete and utter satisfaction, was incredible.

Appa was very impressed with his perseverance and recalled an experience from his own past that had us in splits. Apparently my son's expression mirrored that of one of the movie industry's most respected producers on a night long past, when a similar perseverance had been fuelled by hero worship and a whole load of alcohol.

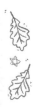

Appa was working on a film whose producer was also a friend—Mr Isari Velan. They had finished a successful shooting schedule in Madurai and were heading back by train. Mr Velan invited Appa over to his coupé for a drink and dinner. The drink before dinner turned into a couple and then more. Two other crewmembers joined them, and they chatted about the movie, congratulating each other on the great shoot and, of course, exchanging the usual movie gossip. It was around midnight when they finally decided to have dinner. The packed food was opened and shared and then everyone got up to go back to their seats. The crewmembers left first and Appa decided to have a final cigarette before retiring to his berth.

Remember, this was the era before smoking was banned and it was normal to light up in private coupés. Although Amma had tried everything to get Appa to stop smoking, nothing had worked so far. An example of how in some cases even perseverance doesn't work! She had finally given in when he promised to smoke with an additional filter. It did not stop her from worrying but she had this notion that the filter would at least help remove some of the nicotine and toxins. Now these filters had to be changed very often and there were always spare ones on him and with his personal staff. But on this particular night he had just one left.

So at midnight and in high spirits, he took out his filter, but as he was fitting it on to the cancer stick, the train jolted and it flew out of his hands. As I said before, this was another era altogether. Trains were not exactly known for comfort, cleanliness or even bright lighting. There would be a few dusty yellow bulbs giving out feeble light that often flickered with the train's speed. So Appa knew it was futile searching for the filter. He just smiled and said, 'There goes my chance to smoke the final cigarette of the night.' It was not just with his hit movie dialogues that Appa kept his word. Once he gave his guarantee about something, it was law. So even though he was a chain smoker, even though the craving for that last cigarette must have been huge, he would not go back on his promise to Amma.

Mr Velan did not give up so easily. He wanted to search for that filter in the dimly lit, cramped space. Appa tried dissuading him by telling him he would smoke when he reached Chennai in the morning, but he was adamant. Fuelled by alcohol, he went on a quest for the elusive last filter. 'I will search for it. The pleasure in doing something when you have the urge for it is special,' he proclaimed before proceeding to go down on all fours and searching for the filter. Appa tried reasoning with him, but he would not relent.

'I would like to try and then say, okay, I'm not able to help you, rather than feel disappointed without trying to help my friend,' he said.

It took almost an hour of scouring the floor on his knees, in that tiny, dark space with dank nooks and crannies that I shudder to even think about, before he emerged victorious, holding aloft the filter. Appa looked on helplessly all this while, but what he remembers most is the childlike glee on Mr Velan's face at that moment of discovery and, of course, the lengths he went to, to fulfil my father's desire.

I can imagine the joy that cigarette gave him.

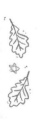

The Making of a Marriage

My life is intertwined with movies. Not that I planned it that way. Just as I had no say in being born into my father's house, my falling in love and marrying an actor were predestined.

I met my future husband at a movie theatre. We were watching *Kadhal Kondein*. At the end of the screening, I spoke to him for the first time and congratulated him, and within a year we were married. I am sure my father had a thousand questions running through his mind when I said, this is the man I want to marry. But my happiness was foremost in my parents' minds and I am happy to say that their confidence was not misplaced. Love and marriage are often a gamble, however carefully thought out they may be, and I was extremely lucky.

Appa, being the conservative father he is, did not want to see his daughter's love life plastered across the pages of newspapers and magazines. He was very clear that there would be no engagement period and the respectable thing to do was to get married. We had a very conventional courtship, very old school. The usual dating rituals did not happen. We called and texted each other a lot, but there were no movie dates or dinners. We never had the chance to meet mutual friends as a couple. We did all that after getting married. We couldn't be seen in public, so when I wanted to meet him, it was always at his home, where we would sit and chat, and most of our time together was spent driving around. Thankfully the ban on dark tints wasn't in effect then; else we would have been discovered before we were ready to admit our relationship. I feel sorry for couples who want to stay hidden today. There is nothing more romantic than driving aimlessly, cocooned from the world outside and certain that no one can look in!

On one of these drives, I was going on and on about our trips to the beach as kids. Of playing near the Gandhi statue, of eating huge meals on the sand, of the freedom that I had taken for granted. I complained about how it was next to impossible for me to go to a beach in Chennai now. He listened quietly and before I knew it, he had driven out of the city and on to East Coast Road. He stopped at a deserted beach and opened the door for me. It was one in the afternoon and the place was steaming under the sun, but I got out, feeling the warm sand under my toes and the gentle breeze trying its best to cool the baking sand. My allergy to the sun forced me back into the car very soon, but I felt a freedom that I had not felt in a long time and I loved the gesture even more.

Our wedding was pretty simple. A traditional engagement was organized the day before the wedding, quite unlike the lavish ceremonies that had become the norm. I was very particular about getting married at home and being blessed by a close gathering of our loved ones. The last thing I wanted was a big fat wedding and Dhanush seemed to find this endearing. So I got married in my father's home, the first one he had bought, amidst the countless happy memories I had of the place.

I count us among the lucky few whose love for each other has deepened in the years after we got married. From love we went to mutual understanding and respect. Like most husbands and wives, we discovered more about each other during the eleven years we have been married, than during our whirlwind courtship. They say women look for their father in their life partner. I had thought of this as some sort of pseudo psychology, until one day the similarities struck me. Being annoyingly adamant about keeping time, for one thing. Which is fine if you are catching a flight, but not when going to have a leisurely meal at a restaurant. (Restaurant managers love us. If we say 7 p.m., we are usually there by 6.55 p.m.) Both my father and my husband are never late for a shoot. If it says 9 a.m., they will be there at 9 a.m. They both have indescribable charisma on screen and a passion for acting. Their work ethic and love for children are just some other traits they share. Thankfully, all great qualities. So all in all, I won in the big marriage gamble. Not that we don't have our ups and downs. Like any other couple, we fight and get mad at each other and then argue and make up and finally compromise. That is what marriage is like between two independent individuals who love each other for what they are, not for who they want them to be.

But marriage did also change things for me, and those around me. For instance, I was never into brands. Appa bought his first luxury car when he was sixty-five. I gifted Amma her first branded handbag on her fiftieth birthday. They just don't understand the concept of buying expensive things for the sake of it. Amma has never bought jewellery for herself in thirty-five years of marriage. I don't think she has entered a jewellery store more than once or twice. I recall a friend of hers saying wistfully, 'If I was a superstar's wife, I would be shopping left, right and centre. Every day!' During our late teens, my mother's idea of shopping was one outing before Diwali. We would visit a sari showroom after working hours to shop for the festival. The other 'shopping' that I enjoyed when I was young was a trip to Nilgiris. It was one of the very few supermarket chains in Chennai. I loved browsing the shelves of ingredients, snacks and more. Amma would buy me a pack of cold flavoured milk for the ride back home. Dhanush spoilt me in this regard. For my first birthday as his wife, he drove all the way to Bangalore to buy me a Louis Vuitton bag. The year after that he gifted me a luxury car. It is hard to go back to my parents' more spartan approach now!

After marriage, I turned into an adult in the eyes of my parents almost overnight. Call it the Indian mentality, or call it the realization by your parents that you are capable of running a household. I did spend most of the early days calling my mother for advice on running a house, taking care of kids or even dealing with the help. Arguments would turn into reminiscences and I finally understood the effort my parents had put into making our lives normal. Since then, my love for them has grown from the blind adoration of a child to a more mature respect for what their lives were like and how they had brought us up irrespective of the pressures. Marrying an actor has given me even more insight into their situation. My husband's companionship has also made me more confident and, of course, he has given me the greatest gift of all—a family of my own. I hope these changes in me have made both Appa and Dhanush proud, not that I would want them to ever discuss it. I shudder to imagine those two perfectionists taking apart my happy-go-lucky attitude to life!

Honeymoon Horrors

Our honeymoon planning established the fact that opposites attract. My idea of a perfect holiday destination is a misty, cool hill station with mountains and forests. Dhanush is a beach person. We were in the process of deciding on a destination when someone mentioned Maldives. A swanky resort had just opened there that everyone was raving about. It was supposedly exotic, luxurious, and the perfect place for newly-weds.

I thought I got quite enough of the sun in Chennai. Moreover, I hate beaches and was not very enthusiastic about lathering myself with greasy layers of sunblock and stocking up on large brimmed hats and umbrellas—and still get fried in the sun. I tan in a second. I have no issues with the colour; I love the beach look, when people come back from their time in the sun looking flushed, happy and healthy. What stops me is my extremely photosensitive skin. Even a little time in the sun has me breaking out in blotchy patches and an outbreak of rashes on every inch touched by the sun. I suffered until I was diagnosed in my teens and from then on I have avoided direct sunlight. This has also caused its share of emotional problems. I used to go out with an umbrella and people thought I was overly concerned about the colour of my skin or that I was a snob, using the umbrella as a shield. I got to hear more than a few snarky comments.

The beach was not my favourite destination for another

reason too. The salt water and sand in every crevice, the waves that literally take the ground from under you, it was all a little too much for me. Certainly nothing like those glossy images of beach resorts and models lounging on the sand make it out to be. So I wasn't very happy about a beach destination, but since I was starting a new life and wanted to try new things, I agreed. Also, Dhanush seemed to hate the cold even more than I hated the sun. The glowing recommendations for the resort also helped.

So here we were, on the brink of an exciting new life together and looking forward to a much needed holiday, although I was still a little apprehensive about the beach. Little did I know that fate had something much worse in store for me and the beach by itself would have been paradise.

Appa was very amused when he heard of our honeymoon destination. He knew my aversion to the sun and the sand and teased me about how marriage could cause such an about-turn in tastes.

As it happened, I fell sick right after the main function. I was advised not to travel and so the Maldives trip was postponed. I had mixed feelings about this, but expected to leave as soon as I had recovered. Meanwhile, a friend of ours from the US flew down to Maldives, expecting us to be there and finding us missing, commandeered our honeymoon suite before we got around to cancelling it. This enterprising friend had an amazing holiday all by himself since his wife and child had headed straight home after the wedding. I was aghast at first but soon saw the funny side of it. And at least the booking didn't go to waste.

By the time I recovered, it was time for Dhanush to start work on an exciting new movie, *Adhu Oru Kana Kaalam*, directed by the legendary Balu Mahendra. Naturally our honeymoon took a back seat. It was a great role for Dhanush and he didn't want to miss out on an opportunity to work with such a stalwart.

He is extremely professional and work comes before anything else. And that's just one of the many qualities that I love about my husband, so I wasn't disappointed at all. In fact, I decided to accompany him for the shoot. Unlike many location shoots of the time, though, this wasn't Switzerland or any naturally beautiful location abroad. It was in Rajahmundry and Dhanush was worried about the amenities at the location. I was still in my post-wedding glow of happiness and too much in love to let him go by himself. Also, I enjoy shoots immensely. Most people are put off by the experience, but I've always found it fascinating, the confusion and scattering of ideas that slowly turn into magic on screen. The thrill of watching a master director at work was the cherry on the cake.

The location in Rajahmundry turned out to be a prison. I am being literal here. It was a real jail! Balu Mahendra wanted authenticity, so the shoot was taking place at a jail with real prisoners lurking in the background. The place we were staying in was the only hotel nearby and was one of the seediest places I have ever been to. I did not want to stay there while Dhanush was away shooting, so decided to accompany him to the location. He told me to stay in the vanity van, but my curiosity got to me and I had to step out. The jail was an experience like no other. I realized that no manufactured set could replicate the atmosphere of that place. I also realized why Balu Mahendra movies are a world apart. A cold shiver passed through me as I entered. Even in broad daylight, it looked eerie. The cast was walking past me in jail uniform and smiled at me as I passed. I smiled back and nodded my head at a few. My husband's makeup man was a few paces behind me; he came running and whispered in my ear. 'Those are not extras dressed as prisoners, they are actual prisoners. Madam, please keep your distance.'

I almost jumped out of my skin in fright.

I had to spend the rest of the shoot waiting at the dingy hotel. I am sure it was quite a difficult time for my new husband. He is one of those actors who gets into the skin of their characters. Not exactly method acting, but he does develop an intense empathy for the role and that is what translates into the intensity that appears on screen. Imagine an actor like that shooting in a jail for scenes that are not exactly stress free, with a celebrated director, and then coming back to a sad, sad hotel room with a bored new wife waiting for him. I was so jobless through the day, I couldn't wait for him to come back and entertain me.

To his credit, he didn't show any irritation. He tried his best to make me comfortable. From replacing all the bedspreads in the room with new ones to getting the entire *Friends* series boxed set for me. The bathroom was the scariest; it almost made me want to run back to the jail. The water heater was an ancient behemoth, right on top of the showerhead. Rust spots covered it and whenever I switched it on, a strange ticking would start. I was pretty sure it was going to explode over my head, right when I was showering. Thankfully the experience didn't last for too long. The shoot was meant to be for two weeks, but the director felt so sorry for us newly-weds that he finished it in a week!

For a little while, I wanted to prove that I could accompany my husband not just to the shopping spots and tourist destinations of the world when it came to shoots, but also to hard-to-live-in places. I got over this notion pretty soon. He stopped asking me to accompany him on shoots away from the city out of sheer dread. Scared of the cribbing he would have to endure if the facilities were bad.

Biography of a Mother

A few kilometres from Theni in southern Tamil Nadu, there is a village called Shankarapuram. A few decades ago a sixteen-year-old girl from the village got married to a twenty-year-old man from another village, five kilometres away. The wedding took place at the Murugan temple in a town called Bodinayakanoor with around hundred people in attendance. It did not exactly start well and maybe that was a portent of the hardships to come. A cousin claimed to be in love with the bride and created a ruckus. He was sent away, after which the wedding proceeded beautifully and perhaps this could be taken as another kind of indication of their future.

She was the fairest in the village and her new husband was a dark, quiet man. They came to the girl's village after the wedding and left the next day for Madurai. She lived in Madurai for two years with her husband and mother-in-law. They were not very well off. Her husband found work in a mill. They had their first child—a son. The delivery was at home, with her husband by her side. She fell ill soon afterwards and he had to quit his job to take care of her and their one-year-old child. Money soon ran out and he had to leave her back in Shankarapuram, while he looked for work. It was not a good time for the young woman, but it was nothing compared to the travails she would have to face in the future. Once married, women were not supposed to go back to their father's home, no matter what the problem, and so she felt unwelcome in her own house.

The husband, meanwhile, took on any work he could find in Madurai. No job was too menial—he had to bring his wife and son back. But two years passed before he could do so. Even then, they weren't together for long. An uncle came to visit and seeing their plight, advised him to look for a job in Madras. He left his wife and son with her parents again and came to the city.

Madras had a vibrant horse-racing tradition and gambling was legal at that point. His uncle got him a job in one of the betting offices that had mushroomed around the city. He took bets and kept the accounts. He wasn't earning enough to bring his wife and child to Madras but he could visit them once in a while and he could send money for their basic expenses. When she became pregnant a year later, he decided to bring her to the city. The village doctor assured them that it was safe for her to travel. They took a train to Madras but on the way she went into labour. Just before they reached Madras, her water broke. The train had to be stopped and they hurried to the nearest hospital, but the baby was born just before they reached. It was a girl. When they finally set foot in the city, they were a family of four, with a baby daughter and a three-year-old son.

That is how my mother-in-law arrived in Madras. It was her first time in any city and there she was, with a newborn and a toddler. It must have been overwhelming. My father-in-law had rented a small place and continued working in the betting shop. She tended to the children and a tiny home on their meagre income.

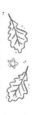

There is one incident she narrated which made me understand the true nature of her struggles. When her first son was four years old, they had to travel to Madurai from her village. Someone had promised my father-in-law a job in Madurai, if he could reach within a certain time. The distance between the two places is close to a hundred kilometres. There was no money to travel even by bus. They had to walk and hitchhike, hoping some good samaritan would offer them a ride, but nobody stopped for them.

After half an hour of walking, the young boy told his mother that he was hungry. She did not know what to do. They had to reach Madurai before they could eat, her child was hungry, and she could do nothing about it. Call it ingenuity, call it the struggle for basic survival, but she calmed him down with a trick. There was a milestone that said ninety kilometres to Madurai. She told him that when they reached a milestone that read eighty kilometres, there would be a shop that sold food and they could eat. When the eighty-kilometre milestone appeared, he asked for food again. She told him the shop seemed to have shifted to the seventy-kilometre milestone. He cried for a bit and then slept on his father's shoulder, too tired to even complain about his hunger. They managed to reach Madurai, walking all the way, taking turns to carry the young child. It is a story that makes me shudder even now. I cannot imagine having to see my child hungry and tired and not be able to do anything about it. It must have been heartbreaking for her.

The family's association with the movies happened by chance. A few movie directors of the time used to visit the place where my father-in-law worked and they suggested he work for them. He quit his job at the betting shop and joined the film industry as an assistant director. Though he worked under the best directors for a few years, his financial situation remained bleak.

My mother-in-law had to make ends meet with a paltry three hundred rupees, month after month. Going hungry herself to feed the kids was a common occurrence. Running the household on a shoestring budget, learning to navigate the city and taking care of the kids must have been quite a task, but she was a fighter. Naïve, yet stubborn enough to survive and do much more than that for her children. A couple of years later, they were blessed with another daughter. My father-in-law climbed a few rungs at work and things started to look a little better, but not much. He still hadn't got an opportunity to direct a movie. The method of payment had also changed. An assistant director was paid Rs 2000 for a full movie. Shoots sometimes went on for six months. My mother-in-law started eating only once a day so that her children could have a full meal at night before they slept. He supplemented his income by transcribing scripts for other directors after work hours. He was paid Rs 300 for each script. Two years later their fourth child was born—a son. The first child that she had in a hospital.

My mother-in-law always did what she thought was best for her children and her kids were at the forefront of every decision she made. Following her instincts, with faith in god and trust in her husband, she fought for survival without succumbing to their abject poverty. And the results were spectacular. She brought up four strong, creative and brilliant individuals who excelled in anything and everything they chose to do. Thankfully things soon started looking up and my father-in-law got a chance to direct a movie.

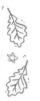

Even in the midst of all the hardship, my mother-in-law would save a coin here and there for her children's education and for her daughters' marriage. She knew that the girls had to be married someday and they would need jewellery. So every penny was saved and there was no eating out or going to movies. There were much more important uses for the money—for her children's future. Her own wishes came last. I admire my mother-in-law immensely and am fascinated by these twin, seemingly opposing traits in her, of strength and sensitivity. If not for her, my husband wouldn't be who he is. And irrespective of her humble background and bitter struggle to survive, she has brought up independent, positive and confident human beings who have made their mark in the world.

My mother-in-law dreamed of her children succeeding academically. She loves her saris and jewellery, but when her first-born joined an engineering college, she sold the jewellery to pay the fees. She had to do the same thing for her second child, who went on to become a doctor. I remember her telling me, it only hurts the first time, when you do it again and again, it doesn't hurt because it is for your children. She wanted her daughters to become doctors and she saw that dream come true. They were told to study well and make it big in life. My sisters-in-law have told me how they never entered the kitchen or learned to cook, as was expected of most girls around them. Their mother told them there would always be time for that later in life.

By the time her second daughter was studying for her post-graduation, her youngest son had started earning some money. He made them proud by paying for her education, even though he had to cut his own short, which is probably her only regret. Dhanush had to join films because no one else was willing to give them dates for a movie. It happened during the last term of his eleventh standard. From what he has told me, Dhanush was a happy-go-lucky boy who wanted to become a chef and travel the world on a luxury cruise liner. He loved movies, but a career in films was not on his radar. Meanwhile, things were not going

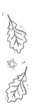

smoothly at home. Financial pressures had mounted and as a final effort, my father-in-law decided to put their money into a single project, hoping it would do well.

Selva, Dhanush's older brother, had written his first script and wanted to direct the movie. It was a coming-of-age story, very different from the usual romances, and they were confident it would do well. The script and the director were ready but no young actor of the time was willing to give them dates. Dhanush's father told him that he had to act in the movie and if he didn't, they would have to abandon the project, pack their bags and leave for Madurai and decide what the future held for them, away from the film industry.

Selva was reluctant to cast his brother, but my father-in-law saw something in Dhanush that nobody else did. He believed that his younger son would make it as an actor. And so the movie was made, though Selva had to give full credit to his more established father as the director to attract distributors. God was kind to them. The movie was a sleeper hit and garnered positive reviews from the critics.

My mother-in-law took to me pretty well. We are stumped by each other's accent at times, but she has always been very open-minded and understanding. The first time I met her was when Dhanush took me home to meet his sisters. His brother and father weren't home but his mother was. She was very cool about it, didn't ask too many questions. I couldn't help but compare it to how my mother would have reacted in the same situation. One question would have followed another and there would have been no respite for the poor visitor.

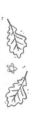

She gave me coffee and delicious cookies. I asked Dhanush about the cookies and he said they had been bought specially for me. They did not want to serve normal biscuits as she thought

I might not like them. From then on my mother-in-law and I have shared a very pleasant relationship. She does not interfere in anything we do and gives us our space and lets us make our own decisions. The only time she complains is when she hasn't heard from us for more than a week. Even then, it is not a matter of the ego at all. She just picks up the phone and calls us for a little chat.

They always say that mothers-in-law cannot love their daughters-in-law as much as they love their daughters. After all, the equation with their son appears to change overnight and the person she thought was her prized possession now lives with someone else. And so she may walk into her son's home with an expression that says, 'It's easy for you now, he is all grown up and well trained!' I think that's quite all right. I am blessed with a mother-in-law who loves me in her own way and I would never compare it with the love she has for her daughters. They have spent their entire life with her. I just walked in a few years ago.

After a certain age, even daughters move out of their homes. It gets a little difficult to live under the same roof, be it daughters or daughters-in-law—given a choice, that is. My mother-in-law realized that we come from totally different backgrounds and she worked around it. I am lucky. A small example is how I am never forced to wear something just because she has bought it for me. I am told to pick what I want, which is so much better than being gifted saris that lie in the wardrobe for years.

When it comes to children too, she encourages me to bring them up exactly as I want to. There is no criticism when it comes to meal choices or the remedies and medication I give them when they are sick, although she herself is paranoid about her health. A headache will have her rushing for a scan; a stomach ache will have her imagining the worst. When it comes to illnesses, she can never think small. Headaches are tumours, a slight fever is the dreaded malaria. It was funny until I realized the reason behind it. She has had people being dependent on her for so long, it has made her anxious about any small symptom that might put her out of commission for a few days. It's her biggest fear. She is petrified of falling ill and being unable to take care of those around her.

As the years pass, our conversations are getting longer and our calls more frequent. We understand each other better, though we haven't done the usual bonding over shopping or cooking. I have to remedy the cooking part because she is an amazing cook and I should learn from her. Her cooking is Dhanush's benchmark when it comes to good food. It is impossible to make him like anyone else's cooking as much, and I have given up the fantasy of finding a cook who can make a meal that tastes like his mother's.

I score the most brownie points from my mother-in-law for my religiosity. I regularly perform pujas at home and she particularly likes my Navaratri pujas. She and my mother come from different communities and though the festivals are the same, the rituals are entirely different. I learned the rituals from my mother and the differences are of great interest to my mother-in-law. She often proudly tells people about this facet of mine.

All four of her children are well settled and living their lives with their own families. It makes her a little lonely, since her entire life revolved around them till recently, yet she accepts it with a smile. She has broken every stereotypical notion I had about mothers-in-law and someday in the future, when I am in her position, I hope my sons' wives feel the same about me.

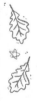

More a Son

A million poets have sought to describe the nature of love and friendship. Novels, stories and plays delve into the complex relationship between mothers and daughters, fathers and daughters, sisters, brothers and everything in between. But strangely, there is very little that comes to mind about fathers-in-law and sons-in-law.

Appa lost his mother when he was seven. He was literally raised by his eldest brother and his wife, who became the mother figure as soon as she married into their family. She raised him alongside her own children and they brought him up like their own son, but I am sure losing his mother at seven left some scars. I have already talked about women looking for their father's qualities in their husbands. I feel (I may be wrong) that one of the factors that attracted Appa to Amma was her nurturing nature. And, in turn, he nurtured her love for her family. From whatever I have heard and seen, I can proudly say that my father was more like a son to her parents than a son-in-law.

My maternal grandparents were very active people. My grandfather worked a regular nine-to-five job till late into his sixties and they drove themselves around quite happily. They had a simple life filled with friends and family. My grandfather would wake up at 5.30 in the morning and go for a walk, come back and

read the newspaper from front to back. The only bad habit he
had was smoking and his heavy addiction caused a heart attack.
He lost a lot of his confidence then and stopped working.

I grew up with them in Bangalore and with me, he insisted on
certain things. One was learning the English language the correct
way. He was the son of a professor of English and had himself
passed out of St. Joseph's College, Trichy. He made me read every
English hoarding we passed on the road and the newspaper every
morning before heading to school. (A very old-fashioned method
of learning, I hated it then, but I realize how helpful it has been
and now make my son do it every morning. He hates it too!)

Grandfather would help with my homework and I can still
recall his beautiful cursive handwriting. It got bigger and bigger
with age as his eyesight failed, but still remained stunningly
precise. Now I see that beauty reproduced only in computer
fonts and rarely by hand. He would also make me write essays
when I visited and would do the same himself, and I still cherish
some of his writing. Vegetarians all their lives, my grandparents
insisted on being 'early to bed and early to rise' and had a zeal for
life that was infectious. I have to thank them for instilling it in
me too.

After a heart surgery that left my grandfather feeling drained,
there was a further bad card that fate dealt us. My grandmother
was diagnosed with cancer. They moved to Madras to be closer
to their children.

My grandmother passed away in her fifty-ninth year. Amma
asked Appa if her father could stay with us, and Appa assented
immediately. There was no hesitation. It would have been the
done thing, especially in those days, for my grandfather to live
with his son, but very naturally and with no uncertainty he came
to his daughter's home. In a society that considers girls as lesser

than boys, partly on the premise that sons would take care of their parents when they got older, Appa showed that it can be the other way round too.

I remember an episode from the nineties, when I was in school. We had planned a holiday to USA and were to leave in a couple of days. It had been decided that my grandfather would stay back home due to concerns about his health. A day before we were to leave, though, Appa walked into the room where my sister and grandfather were playing Scrabble. He pulled out an envelope and handed it to my grandfather. It contained his passport and tickets for him to join us for the holidays. I remember the expression on my grandfather's face. It was beautiful. All Appa did was to pat my grandfather on the shoulder and say, 'Pack your bags, we are going to America.'

It was a memorable trip. We visited Disneyland and Universal Studios. At most of the rides there were notices that prohibited heart patients from boarding, among other warnings. Amma would not get on the tamest rides, but Appa and my grandfather (much to my mother's concern) would grin and get on the rides like ten-year-olds. Appa would assure Amma, 'I am there, and he is enjoying himself. Your father will not get hurt. This is good for him.' We managed to drag my mother on to one ride just once, and I remember she chanted and screamed almost every god's name in the Indian pantheon before it ended. We laughed ourselves silly. And Appa was right; it did my grandfather a whole lot of good.

Around the year 2000, my grandfather's age started catching up with him. He was losing his memory and his mobility. It was around the same time that Dhanush and I had started talking about a future together. I knew in my heart that he was the one I was going to marry, and I wanted my grandfather to be around for it. Would my future husband understand that? I told him about it and the universe showed me once again that my choice was right. He agreed, and that was the main reason we had such a quick wedding. It turned out to be the right decision. Grandfather blessed us and even recognized that the man before him was his grandson-in-law. And only a year later, he was gone. Appa lost a father figure that year and gained a son.

I am biased about my life partner, and there are a zillion incidents I could document about him, but this one is etched in my heart forever. One of the most difficult times in my life was when Appa fell sick. I was at the hospital the entire time and zoned out every other facet of my life. It was all about his treatment, his recovery and his comfort. I am sure anybody who has had a sick parent can relate to this. Husband and children took a back seat. I was so high-strung that people avoided me. When we had to travel to Singapore for further treatment, my sister and I took turns at the hospital. It was not our home country and the simple things we took for granted in Chennai took time and effort here, particularly at the hospital. Amma also was not well and was too distraught to be at Appa's bedside.

We were there for three months, living out of suitcases. The hospital took up all our time. I just could not be a daughter and a mother at the same time. All my mind space was taken. My husband is a self-made man, his work ethic is famous, and by then he was doing really well, due to his hard work and god's grace. (He never used my father's connections or my pedigree to get ahead. In fact, he once mentioned in an interview that it undermined his hard work, when people assumed his success was due to his family and his in-laws.) That year he was doing three movies, which entailed crazy timings, hundreds of people dependent on his schedule, not to mention large sums of money at stake. It was a big deal for a young actor, but I could not even think beyond the hospital walls. I dumped the kids with him. He had come to Singapore to drop us off and make sure everything was arranged right, but I wouldn't let him go back to India to shoot. I needed someone to stay some nights at the hospital. My sister and I just couldn't handle it by ourselves. Amma would stay with the kids.

Being from a film family, I could almost see the flashback in my head. My Amma approaching Appa about her father; me approaching my husband about mine. A split screen appears. History repeats itself. And like most Indian movies, mine had a happy ending too (despite some heartache for the producers). Dhanush stayed.

It was not just the extra hands in a foreign country that helped. The emotional support was tremendous. We could, as a family, concentrate on getting Appa better. My husband became a true son to Appa in those three months, staying up with him so that I could sleep, keeping him company, and his spirits up.

And don't worry about the producers. He compensated them amply for their patience and I am happy to say that all three films were hits at the box office and all was well in the end, including Appa's health!

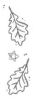

The Sacred Thread

Black, red, yellow and even green. On the left foot if you are a girl, right if you are a guy. Wrist, neck, waist, arms, no part of the body is spared.

Some habits are integral to our childhood, even though we have no idea why. There were always a few threads from a variety of temples, dargahs and other places of worship that adorned my ankles and wrists. A friend or relative would make the trip and return with some prasad and a thread, which would end up tied around our wrists or ankles. Some were for health, others to ward off the evil eye or for prosperity, and some to prevent nightmares. I have tried to ask a number of people about their significance, but was never satisfied with the answers. (Yes, I have Googled them too!)

Some of the explanations were downright ridiculous. One old aunt said that a black thread tied around a young girl's ankle helped keep her fertile. Why a young, unmarried girl needed to be fertile was a question that occurred to me only after she passed away. A family priest was obsessed with these threads, and we got to hear many tall tales that explained the history of each thread that he collected from temples across India. Every one of them was holy according to him and some had lockets with the images of gods attached to them. He came with these and

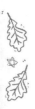

went away after accepting a dhoti or some money for his efforts. If he had his way, every piece of thread that was manufactured would be blessed. He also believed that there was a particular time for bathing, for eating, for sleeping etc., that he followed, all according to some ancient superstitions.

Such attitudes are not limited to India. I remember a story that a friend once told me about a man from Philippines who was given a sacred thread to tie around his neck by a holy man. The man's mother died a few days after that and he believed that the thread had caused all the bad karma he had gathered to transfer to his mother, who then proceeded to die, leaving him cleansed. I was shocked at the interpretation and even more shocked to hear that the man continued to wear the thread, thinking it was highly effective.

I am a scaredy cat, I must confess, when it comes to sleeping alone and in the dark, and these threads often gave me a sense of security when I was younger, so I never entirely discounted them. I had a red thread around my wrist, which was supposed to help ward off evil spirits. I wore it in my teens, and then one day decided it was just a crutch and wanted to do away with it. It took me a year to get over my psychological dependence on that thread, but eventually I realized that I could sleep peacefully without it too. And just like that, it went back to being a little red thread from a powerful talisman that I thought I was dependent on. The thread works on a person's mind, making them feel a little braver, a little more confident. The danger begins when you start attributing all your success to it.

Confession time—I still have a black thread tied around my left ankle, which is supposed to ward off the evil eye. Not that I believe in it, but the nostalgia and comfort in retaining something from my childhood make me continue the tradition. Appa also has one around his right ankle, and when I asked him about it, he shrugged and said that he'd had one since he could remember and he had never questioned it. I could see a reflection of my own sense of continuity in that answer. When someone ties a thread for you, it's not just plain old superstition. It's a testament of love: I love you and care for you, but I know I cannot protect you from every bad thing, real or imagined, so I would like to keep this token somewhere on you, to give you and myself comfort.

Certainly, that is what I mean when I continue with the custom. Both my sons wear a black thread around their ankles, which I hope reminds them of our love for them. Someday they are bound to question the practice and decide for themselves whether they want to wear it or not—and I am fine with that.

Weighty Matters

What goes around comes around. For those of you who have children, you know the cycle of recurring moments that involve you, your children and your parents.

If Appa is simple in his eating habits, Amma is extravagant. She loves feeding people. I loved eating and she loved feeding me when I was a kid. Almost everything was drenched in butter and ghee, and I had not even heard of carbs. Sweets and savouries were made at home without skimping on any ingredient, however fattening. We ate mostly home-cooked food and even when we ate out, pizzas, burgers, sugar-heavy drinks and refined zero-nutrient snacks were not on the menu, for they were yet to find their way to Madras. I always ate heartily and was active; Amma was happy. I wasn't obese, but I was bigger than most children my age.

I can't be as easy-going with my kids as she was with hers. Junk food is everywhere and the temptations are greater. But all my best intentions go down the drain when I stay with Amma, who still insists on filling us up with the richest food at every opportunity. My usual break at home consists of eating, chatting with Appa and sleeping. Amma takes care of the boys, relishing the time spent with them. One such evening, she had prepared fluffy golden puris accompanied by yummy chana, garnished with freshly cut onions. Appa, the boys and I were eating while she served us. My older son sat on a chair next to us at the table while the younger one was perched on the table as he was still too small to reach it from a chair. Now Yatra loves fried things, like most kids, and these 'straight from a vat of oil' puris were heaven for him. As he was about to reach for his fourth one, I asked him to stop. The fried puris and accompanying spicy gravy were not good for him to indulge in so late in the evening. I told him to end his meal with something light—a glass of milk or a few mouthfuls of rice and curd. He was obviously disappointed and tried his best heart-melting gaze on me, but I was adamant.

Appa is not so strong, especially when it comes to his grandchildren. He immediately placed another puri on the child's plate and said, 'Yatra, take one more ... I'll ask your mother's permission for it ... She won't say no.' Yatra looked at me for confirmation. I knew that if I said no, I would look like the tyrant mommy who said no to food that he thought was yummy (didn't plan for that to rhyme!). So, unhappily, I nodded at him and stared daggers at Appa. Once the kids had left, Appa in his usual calm manner tried to convince me that children should never be stopped from eating. There is a saying in Tamil that a young stomach can digest even a stone. But I was not ready to give up and as the conversation progressed, I realized my mother was standing quietly, listening to us with a smile on her face. Usually, when it came to anything to do with food, she would jump in and contribute her own philosophy, which can be best described as 'feed till they are full and then some more!'

Her silence was so out of character that I mentioned it to Appa, saying something was seriously wrong with Amma, she wasn't coming to her grandchildren's rescue as she usually did. He turned to her and asked for her support. After all, she was well known for shouting at friends, relatives, even strangers, if they said anything about kids overeating.

She shook her head. 'When she was the same age as Yatra is now, you had the same argument with me about her overeating the exact same thing.' Appa immediately recalled the incident and you should have seen the sheepish expression on his face!

I don't remember it, but apparently I was doing the same thing at lunch one day and Appa was looking at me worriedly. He has very basic food requirements and I guess he just couldn't understand my gluttony. Amma noticed him watching me and chided him for it. She thought he was being cruel, but Appa was worried that the world could be a cruel place if I ended up being fat. I was already a chubby kid, and he must have been worried about the bullying I would be subjected to. I gather even marriage prospects were mentioned in the course of that conversation. Amma had gone on to place before him the same arguments that he offered to me when I stopped Yatra from overindulging. As the argument continued, I had rather opportunistically reached for another puri. Appa stopped me, and Amma snapped. She said to him, 'There will come a time when you regret this and beg her to eat!'

I eventually grew out of the baby fat and once school activities, tennis, dance, etc., gathered momentum, it became a constant struggle to actually find time to keep myself well fed. I remember Amma begging me to have another sip before I rushed out and Appa asking me to take one more bite when we went out to eat.

It had come almost full circle now, and I realized why Appa was being so adamant. I was happy that Amma had not contributed to the worry about my size, but I understood Appa's point of view as well: society does not look favourably upon bigger-sized people, especially women. I had to tread a fine balance between urging my children to eat healthy while not contributing to a bad body image. And of course, grandparents will be grandparents. So, just as it is my job to control the children's excesses, it is theirs to indulge those same extravagances.

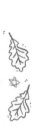

Kiddy Lessons

Family holidays were a big occasion for us when we were kids, and I love to continue the tradition with my own children, though it can be a little tough. At home, I have help with most things. The clothes are washed and ironed, the cook takes care of breakfast, lunch and dinner and all I have to do is make sure the children eat, play and sleep on time. Which I insist happens according to a strict timetable.

I can be quite the stickler for routine, almost dictatorial in my need for obedience (my sons, if asked, could supply you with a whole load of other unflattering terms, I am sure). I am convinced that growing children need their sleep, and although I may sound like a nagging granny, I cannot stress its importance enough. Left to them, sleep would be the last priority. They think it is a waste of valuable playtime and as they get older, it's harder to make them stick to their bedtime. So a holiday abroad is a bribe that's dangled throughout the school year. I couldn't do this when they were young. (Double toddler nightmares and international flights do not mix!) I imagined every horrible scenario, including losing them in a vast theme park, running around frantically searching for them, while they sat back in some hiding place, watching me and laughing as I went crazy! (I must also admit I was not taken by the prospect of bathing, feeding, putting to sleep and ensuring all-day entertainment for the twin terrors, all by myself.) So it was only four years ago that I finally got to take them on a holiday.

Now I have been on flights where children have wreaked havoc. Running up and down the aisle, screaming. Jumping over people, stepping on their legs, hitting their shins. The worst was a nine-hour flight where a toddler wailed throughout. The mother tried everything she possibly could, the flight attendants tried, the people in the neighbouring seats tried, but the child just went on wailing. For nearly nine hours straight. (He wasn't sick, probably just bored and irritated.) My kids have been kind to me. They usually take a short nap or watch the inflight entertainment. Thank god!

The first such trip we went on was to Hong Kong. Not too far, nor too close. It had a Disneyland, which we visited almost as soon as we landed. To be perfectly truthful, I enjoyed it even more than the boys did. I felt like a princess! I wore a tiara, took photographs with every character who crossed my path and generally had a whale of a time. I am sure I embarrassed the boys and if it had gone any further (they did not have a Snow White costume in my size) they would have abandoned me then and there, refusing to acknowledge that I was their mother.

Children love repetition. I can almost see the parents among you nodding their heads, thinking of those bedtime sessions when you were forced to read the same book or sing the same lullaby again and again and again. So it should come as no surprise that our next holiday abroad was to Disneyland in Hong Kong. The weather was lovely and it was Christmas time. The kids were a bit more grown up and could enjoy the rides and since they were familiar with the place, there was no running around to find Mickey or Goofy. My husband was also able to get a few days

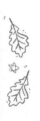

off and that made the whole trip very special. We love planning trips as a family, but when you combine a busy actor husband and the school calendar, it is difficult. We hate them missing out on vacations, so I usually take them, but having their father around is, of course, the tops. I still remember how gleefully they watched the parade with their father and how the colourful lights from the fireworks reflected off their excited faces.

The summer after that, we asked them where they wanted to go for their holidays.

The answer was, 'Disneyland!'

I put my foot down and luckily their father had a shoot in London that year and I was able to convince them that visiting their Appa on location was an exciting prospect. They ended up having a good time and eventually gave up cribbing about missing Disneyland and its wonders.

But the summer after that, there was no escape. I was done with Mickey and the gang and had grown out of my desire to be princess for a day (and they did not have a costume in my size, remember?). The kids put their foot down this time and begged, pleaded, cajoled and convinced me into doing a third trip. My husband gave in first. 'They love it so much, and in a few years they will grow out of it. So why not indulge them?'

Yatra was at the questioning stage of childhood. 'Where is the kitchen on a plane? Why is it a pressure cabin? Who drives the plane when the pilot is eating? If it is on autopilot, why do we need a pilot at all? What is time difference? If they can serve chocolate cake, why can't they serve strawberry too? Is Mickey real?' He wouldn't settle for my brief answers (so that I could get back to that much needed nap) and didn't give up until he had a logical answer that satisfied him.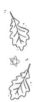

This questioning was accompanied by a radically contrary

habit of claiming independence from his mother. 'I know how to put on the seatbelt, you don't have to help me, Ma! I can go to the bathroom by myself. I can get my own boarding pass. Please let me carry my own passport, I am big enough, I won't lose it.'

I can tell you, running down the aisles and screaming seemed like a good option that day.

So we landed in Hong Kong and went straight to the hotel where we had stayed three times already in five years. By now the staff there knew us by sight. The concierge even complimented me on my weight loss. (I know. It's his job to butter up the guests.) We checked in and the boys started running about, which did not bother me much as there were fifty other kids doing the same thing around us. Obviously they were hyper excited and wanted to go to the park immediately. Realizing that if I refused, all that extra energy would be used to torment me, I agreed. So we took off, to the same rides, the same attractions, greeted the same characters. I realized I could lead an alternate life as a Disney tour guide. But I gradually started enjoying it. The place is so lovely and positive that you cannot help but smile. There were families of all sizes and kids of all ages having a wonderful time. Of course there were a few wailers and bawlers. Some because they wanted extra cotton candy, others scared when a human-sized Donald Duck waddled towards them.

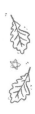

Yatra decided it was the perfect time to assert his independence even further. I lectured them constantly on the need to stick together but he would run ahead of us every time. He knew the place well, so he figured he could get away with it. I would get anxiety attacks every time he ran away from me into the crowds but he would just not listen. I was frazzled by the constant need to remind him, while keeping an eye on Linga. Horror stories about lost kids plus the fact that a few people had recognized us made me paranoid. It's better to be safe than sorry, my own sheltered childhood had taught me that. We stopped at a candy truck, loaded ourselves with every sugary confection that met the eye, and were waiting to pay for it when Yatra spotted an ice-cream truck, which he wanted to raid immediately.

I asked him to wait until I had finished paying, but Mr Independent decided to run ahead. He had a little money on him and, with a cocky air, instructed us to join him when we were done. It wasn't too far away, so I could trace his path to the truck, and I saw him buy the ice cream and turn around. I couldn't resist it. Towing the younger one behind me, I quietly hid behind the truck and waited. At first he waited for us to join him, then he took tentative steps around the truck. Finally he came back to the candy truck, looked around and still couldn't find us. I could see the growing panic in his eyes. The jaunty air was gone and he started calling out for his mom. Tears flowed down his cheeks as he became increasingly desperate. The little boy who wanted his mom was back. My heart sank. Feeling terrible, I ran to him, hating myself, and gave him a hug. Between sobs and the tightest hug I had ever received from him, he said, 'I was just putting on an act for you, Amma, I wasn't scared at all. I was trying to scare you!'

All I could do was kiss his blotchy face and enjoy the hugs and kisses while they lasted. A darker part of me hoped he had learned his lesson.

Tough Love

One relationship that has taken me by surprise is the one I share with my brother-in-law, Selvaraghavan. I never realized he would go from barely speaking to me to becoming my mentor.

The first time he spoke with me was over the phone and he didn't know who was at the other end. It happened when Dhanush and I had just started getting to know each other and were constantly chatting on the phone. Dhanush was travelling with Selva, who noticed his brother clinging to the phone, texting furtively and disappearing to make calls, even going into the bathroom with the phone. When he asked him about his sudden love affair with the phone, Dhanush avoided the question. One day Dhanush came into the room, talking on the phone, and fell on the couch next to Selva, who kept staring at him. Dhanush pointedly ignored him and kept talking. I'm sure it was some good-natured brotherly teasing.

'So who is this girl you were talking to?' Selva asked once Dhanush had put the phone down.

'You know it's a girl, right? Now let it be.'

Selva kept staring at him.

'It's my girlfriend.'

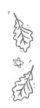

Selva was stunned into silence, but it didn't last long. He started a relentless campaign to find out who it was. At first he thought it was the actress who was working with Dhanush at that point. Then suspicions fell on anyone even remotely connected with Dhanush in the past. Then he fell to investigating friends and their friends. Nobody knew anything. He came up with nothing and it was killing him.

One afternoon, while they were together in a car, Dhanush's phone rang and he picked it up. Selva announced that he wanted to say hello to the girl who had captured his brother's heart. Dhanush asked me if it was okay, and I said yes. He passed the phone to his brother.

Selva: 'Hi.'

Me: 'Hi.'

Selva: 'So, how are you doing?'

Me: 'I'm good, thank you, and you?'

Selva: 'Yeah, fine. So what is your name?'

Me: 'Aishwaryaa.'

Selva: 'Hmm. Just Aishwaryaa... not Aishwarya Rai or Rajinikanth?'

Me: 'Rajinikanth, actually.'

There was silence for a moment, then Selva hung up and turned to Dhanush.

Dhanush: 'What? Did she hang up?'

Selva: 'No, I did. She said she is Aishwaryaa Rajinikanth. I think I heard it wrong.'

Dhanush: 'No, you didn't.'

My brother-in-law nearly jumped out of his skin. At first he thought Dhanush was pulling a fast one, then he got excited and then worried.

Selva: 'This is Rajinikanth. Will he send goons to bash up my little brother?'

Dhanush: 'Ha ha… yes, if this were a movie.'

Selva finally calmed down enough to feel embarrassed about disconnecting the phone and asked Dhanush to call me.

I, on my part, hadn't called back because I didn't know what was happening. I just thought he was being rude, because he disapproved of our relationship. When the phone rang again, it was Selva.

'Hi again. I'm sorry I hung up like that. You guys just took me by surprise.'

So that was my introduction to my brother-in-law.

Whenever we met after that, he would nod his head, not make much eye contact, maybe say a quick hello and walk off. I don't think he spoke a complete sentence to me during that period. When I asked Dhanush, he just told me to let him be. He is a reserved person, I was told, and takes time to warm up to people. By the time I was married and came into the house, he had moved out, so I didn't get to see much of him. I did hear from the staff at the house that he would enquire about my well-being whenever he came home and asked everyone to make sure I was comfortable. I found that very sweet.

Once, Dhanush had to go for a shoot in Hyderabad for two months and I accompanied him. This was some time after our wedding. The movie was being directed by Selva and by then he had spent enough time with me for us to get along splendidly. I found him to be one of the most creative people I had met. He has a quirky personality and a completely out-of-the-box way of seeing things. I would often wonder how he came up with a scene or a situation in a movie. I loved sitting and chatting with him

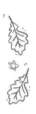

and we had some fun conversations throughout the shoot. The movie was *Pudhupettai* and it turned out to be a path-breaker. It portrayed the unglamorous side of criminal life, a rarity in Tamil cinema, with a flawed and dark protagonist played by Dhanush.

It helped that Selva would always take my side when I had a tiff with Dhanush. He always made sure I was comfortable and looked after. He had a girlfriend who would get annoyed at times because he was being so attentive to me. I happened to overhear his reply to this complaint and it endeared him even more to me.

He said, 'She comes from a totally different background and she has never seen any hardship. I don't want it to happen after she has married into our family. I feel protective about her as an elder brother.'

Most of our conversations were about movies and he would often ask me when I was going to make my own film. A year or so later, he came home from a shoot in Hyderabad and we were having dinner when conversation turned to my career. I told him that maybe it was time I looked out for work as an assistant director before working on a script for myself. My son had turned three and he could be left with family for a part of the day. He listened patiently and that same evening, before we turned in for the night, he asked me to pack my bags and leave for Hyderabad with him. I refused, unable to even think of leaving my baby alone for two weeks. But Selva had already spoken to Dhanush and my mother about it. They would take turns looking after the baby. Selva was upset that I hadn't thought of him in the first place and was looking around for work. He did not see any reason why I should work for someone else when there was a director in the family, who was making a movie right at that moment.

I made excuses. How would Dhanush handle running the house? How would my toddler fare without me? Selva put his foot down. He told me that everyone could take care of themselves when they were required to. Nobody was dependent on anybody. Since you take it upon yourself to do all these things, it's become a habit for everyone, but if you are away, they will form new and independent habits, he said. Everyone had the right to pursue their dreams and if I really wanted to become a director, I should be willing to prioritize and take decisions accordingly, else I would be sitting at home and taking care of people for the rest of my life.

I was still undecided. He left with an ultimatum. Either show up for the morning flight or never speak to him about it again. This was the last time he was giving me the opportunity. I ran to Dhanush for advice. He urged me to go. My mother was ecstatic about having her grandson for two weeks and Selva had already promised to let me travel to Chennai during the breaks in the shoot. Excited, nervous and unable to sleep, I decided I was going to do it.

I took the flight to Hyderabad and we drove to the film city where the shoot was to take place and where we would be staying for the next two weeks. The movie was *Ayirathil Oruvan*. He put me up in a room next to him and made sure I was comfortable. The next day we had to go scout for locations and make decisions about the shoot, which was going to start the day after. I was a bit rusty, it had been years since I was on the groundwork team. The first and last time I had worked as an assistant before this was for my father's movie, *Baba*, directed by Suresh Krishna. It was not much of an experience, I must say. I was more of an observer; no one would let me do any work. I managed to learn just two things—how to work a clapboard and how to write an edit report. The team would just shake their heads and say, 'Ma'am, you don't need to do this, you just watch and we'll do it

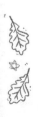

for you.' I did learn a lot just by being on the set every single day and following the director around, but I did not have any hands-on experience.

With Selva, the first day was almost similar. I went along with him and the team. There were two cars. I travelled in the car with him and when the day's work was done, we left together for the hotel where we were staying. A little while later, he called and asked me to have dinner with him and during the meal he outlined what he wanted me to do. I needed to be at the shooting spot an hour before he came in. The only perk I would have is that I would be staying at the hotel in the room next to his, which was for my safety. I would travel with the other ADs, work with them, eat with them, and leave when they left. I would not be treated any differently. This was a different man sitting in front of me. Not my brother-in-law, but the director I was working under. It was a bit of a jolt for me, this difference in tone, but it felt good that he was taking me seriously, and I agreed.

The next morning, I am ashamed to say that I overslept and was ready only when Selva was leaving the hotel. I apologized and told him it wouldn't happen again, but he didn't take it very well. He gave me a stern warning and was quite scary as he did so. When we reached the shoot, he became an entirely different man, a taskmaster in every way, and by the end of the day, I realized this wasn't going to be a cakewalk for me. The next couple of weeks were going to be tough. Marriage had made me pretty laid-back and everything happened around me according to my convenience, but this was a different ballgame. I was working for one of the most demanding directors in the field, who treated me exactly as he would any other newcomer on the set. I even got yelled at like the others. But there was one advantage. In the evening, after the shoot, I could pick his brains and try and get him to explain why he was being so difficult. It was simple, really. He wanted me to toughen up.

'The movie industry isn't an easy place to work in. It's a man's world and if you want to get work done, you need to be tough as nails.'

What he meant was on a movie set a woman needs to assert herself—only then will people treat her with respect.

'People have to take you seriously and in order for that to happen, you have to toughen up. I will yell if you are slow or make mistakes. There is no place for ego or hurt feelings when you are learning. You are in a school that shows no mercy. I am not going to be soft on you because of who your father is, or because you are family. You are my assistant on the set and that's it. If you can't handle it, you are still welcome on the set as my sister-in-law, but you will learn nothing. But if you want to pursue this as a career, this is how you will be treated. You did not leave your child at home and come here to fool around. You have dreams and they can only come true if you are willing to put in the effort. If you move on to directing a film, it should be due to merit, not because of your family. If I have a daughter, this is what I would wish for her and this is how I would treat her.'

Every word he said hit home. I understood what he was doing and why. It was because he really cared for me and respected me. I took him seriously then, and that was when my real learning began. I extended my stay.

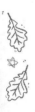

A couple of weeks later, I was late again. The previous day's shoot had been incredibly taxing and I had got only a couple of hours of sleep. I texted Selva saying I just couldn't get out of bed and would love to have an extra hour to rest. I asked whether I could leave with him, just for that one day. I didn't get any reply. I dozed off and the car left without me. The shooting spot was about two kilometres from the hotel. When I got ready and asked for the car, the manager told me that the director had instructed that no car should be sent back to the hotel to pick me up. I was very upset. It was only the second time in the entire schedule that I was late.

I walked to the shooting spot and it was half past eight by the time I reached. Selva had already arrived. The shoot was to begin at 9 a.m. and I hurried to my tasks for the day, but another AD stopped me. He said he had been instructed by the director not to let me on to the set that day. I was shocked. Everyone was getting on with their work as I stood at the periphery of the shoot. After an hour Selva walked out of the vanity van and onto the set. He saw me but did not say a word. I ran after him and requested him to let me in. He turned to one of the assistants and said, 'If I get to know that anyone of you has given her something to do or even spoken to her, you will be sent back home right away.'

I was aghast, but my ego did not let me give up. I stood there from 9 a.m. to 6 p.m. The production boy kept bringing me food and coffee, but I refused to eat or drink. I was extremely angry and upset. Selva had taken things too far. He was being unnecessarily mean and rude and it was just too much. I refused to budge from the spot and nobody dared approach me, they knew they would get fired. When the shoot wrapped up, I got into the team car and was dropped at the hotel. I didn't even want to see Selva's face. I called Dhanush, hoping he would sympathize, but he told me that his brother had called and told him not to interfere in the matter. I hung up on him angrily.

A while later there was a knock on my door. I opened it to find Selva standing outside. I was so angry, I wanted to slap him. He asked if he could come in. I let him in silently and he sat down without saying a word. The humiliation came rising up and I wanted to shout and rant at him, but before I could say anything, he asked me if I had eaten. I said no and he got up to order room service.

'Never take your anger out on your stomach; nothing is going to change if you starve yourself. It's a very silly way of expressing anger.'

He sat me down then and told me that the incident had hurt him too, but he had big dreams for me.

'I was disappointed that you were making excuses and still wanting things to be flexible. That is not what I would expect of my own child. That is not what is expected of Rajinikanth's daughter. You should be an example. If anyone says that this girl takes things easy because of her family and wonders why you are doing all this if you aren't serious about it, it would hurt me and I know it would hurt you. I have scared you and taught you a lesson. I know you will never be late again.'

After that day, I continued to work with the team until the film was completed.

Who would have thought that I would become so close to Selva and eventually consider him my mentor? Nobody could have predicted that my usually reserved brother-in-law would take me under his wing and prepare me for the hard realities of life in the movie industry. They say relationships evolve every day. What better example than Selva and I?

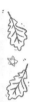

A Few Hours at the Shooting Spot

It is my husband's directorial debut. It has been his dream to direct a movie someday and now it's coming true. We are all very excited. I have read the script, seen its inception, and I love it. The story is endearing and different from what's happening at the moment in south Indian cinema. The first look has released to a lot of interest, both from the industry and the public. I go to the shooting spots as often as I can to observe how he functions as a director. I love watching the action and have learned something new every time I visit. Today the shoot is taking place at my in-laws' house. I rush over after work. It's two birds with one stone: I can watch the shoot and spend some time with my mother-in-law. She doesn't seem very perturbed by the intrusion. After all, her husband and eldest son are already in the ranks of Tamil cinema's renowned directors. Now her youngest son is continuing the legacy.

I walk in and the energy is amazing. Imagine a wedding hall a few minutes before the ceremony is to take place. The entire day at a shooting spot runs on a similar energy. All these characters before you, amusing, irritating, interesting, brilliant, all working in a frenzy towards a single goal of transforming an idea into a movie. Since I've come straight from work, I have my laptop with me. I sit on the sidelines of the chaos and jot down what I see.

Long iron beams are mounted on the ceiling, all over the house. They support the lights and other equipment. All the fans and hanging lights have been dismantled. The scene is being shot in the living room, which looks totally different. The furniture has changed; a four-seater has replaced the eight-seater dining table. The drapes have been changed too. The sofas are different, and all this has happened overnight. Sprawling lengths of black cloth are all over the place. They are used to cut the glare from the overhead lights or to cover light coloured items. They are also at times used on the floor, a carpet of black cotton. I see cameras, light stands, cutters (also used to cut the glare) and around them, a sea of people that includes the cast, the crew, the assistants, members of the unit and various hangers-on.

Two children catch my attention. A boy of around nine and a girl of about six. The boy seems like a professional, mature beyond his years. He is very comfortable on set and knows why he is here and what he needs to do. The confidence is apparent on his face and he behaves like a veteran with numerous movies under his belt. He talks very little, comes to the shot when called, does his part and then retires to his seat and concentrates on his PlayStation. The girl is a handful. The assistant directors are having a hard time with her. She talks nineteen to the dozen and is running all over the place. Exactly at the moment that she is needed for a shot, she disappears, although they find her pretty quickly thanks to her non-stop chatter. It's apparent that it is her first time on set, but her face is full of mischief that could translate very well onscreen. The mother is trying to get her to follow instructions but the kid doesn't care. When she needs to be serious in front of the camera, she bursts out in giggles. She

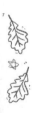

just wants to have fun. Nobody minds too much because she is cute. Most of the time, the mothers of both children stand in a corner, immersed in their phones. They take calls now and then and appear to be at ease with their surroundings.

The senior actors' assistants hover around their bosses. They tend to their every need, from carrying the touch-up kit, mirror, water, to getting beverages and meals to suit the actor's taste. If the shoot is outdoors, they are often seen holding an umbrella over the actor's head. They all carry a similar kind of bag—a black one, the length of a laptop bag but much wider, with a long strap—and they carry it till the end of the shoot. It is like a symbol of their profession. None of them will part with it even for a second.

Some assistants stand next to the actors and hold their phones while the scene is being shot and hand them back once the director yells cut. The actors trust only their assistants to hold on to these. The other option is to leave the phone or iPad in the vanity van, which, of course, is unthinkable. People do not want to be parted from their digital devices for a second longer than is absolutely necessary. Though I must say, I have also seen some actors who prefer books to gadgets.

While the shooting is in progress, the assistants form a gang in a corner, murmuring to each other, eyes constantly on their bosses. As soon as the shot is done, they rush towards the actors. Phone, makeup kit, water, mirror, anything the actor needs is a glance away. I have also seen them act as gatekeepers when the actor is inside the vanity van. No one is allowed to enter without permission. The only outsider allowed is the assistant director sent to call the actor for the shot. The assistants usually travel everywhere with their bosses and are often the first ones to take and post a selfie from the location. I have seen a few ask the set photographer to take shots of them posing diligently with the phone or another assistant.

Successful actors' assistants are the most spoilt of the lot. They usually have their own assistants, who do all the running around. Their main job is to interpret the star's wants and dislikes and dispatch the junior assistants to take care of them. The hero or heroine wants a cup of green tea, the main assistant will ask the junior to get it with enough drama to alert the entire set. The junior will scamper away and come back with a cup, then hand it over to the main assistant, who hands it to the star with a bow and a flourish. It's extremely entertaining to watch. The higher the actor is on the popularity scale, the more dramatic the assistant's performance is. The actors themselves do not create much of a fuss. In fact, the assistants get even more pompous when the actors are not around and sometimes create unnecessary distractions. Of course, this is not true of all stars or their assistants.

Then there are the production assistants, who are just the opposite. Discreet and constantly moving around with something useful in their hands. On a commercial movie set there are usually six to ten production assistants. The most wanted one is the guy in charge of refreshments. It is his job to keep the set well fed, alert and on their toes. He usually has flasks of tea or coffee, jugs of buttermilk and lemonade, paper cups and bottles of water on him, depending on the time of the day. He is constantly serving food or drink to the crew. One comes up to me and asks if I need anything. He knows my choices by now. He served me green tea half an hour back and I know he will be back in another half hour to check on me again. I often judge the efficiency of the production unit by how well the production assistant keeps the unit fed and caffeinated!

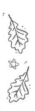

The other production assistants handle the rest of the crew. The more experienced ones are usually with the cinematographer and the director. The rest are distributed throughout the unit, some with the cast and some with the crew.

Another busy job is that of the cameraman's assistant. He has to be on his toes all the time. The AD can take a break while the cameraman is working. The actors' assistants get a break while the shoot is taking place. But a cameraman's assistant has to adjust the lighting after every scene and prepare for the next scene. It's not an easy job. Moving the heavy lights, snaking the cables around the spot and finding which cable connects to what, and then connecting everything to the electrical board without frying us all. The angle and intensity of each light sometimes require to be adjusted eight to ten times in each scene and they have to do all the shifting by hand. But these are hardy men who scoff at electric shocks and work with immensely hot and heavy lights. I have even seen them work during meal breaks, gulping down their food before setting up the scene so that it is ready by the time the cast and the rest of the crew finish their lunch or dinner. I am sure they don't even know what's going on in the film, the story, or even the scene they are setting up. The lights, stands, skimmers, cutters, cables, boards and black cloth are what their jobs revolve around.

I spot a new AD. It's easy; he looks like he is just out of school—and rather lost. He has absolutely no clue what is going on and nobody is taking the time to explain anything to him. Time is money and he will have to learn the ropes himself. He cannot sit down, or people will think he is not interested. He can't just stand around because he'll get in the way of the crew who are actually working. He walks around, trying to look busy, trying to be helpful, but he is either rebuffed or ignored. He runs along with the rest of the ADs when the director gives instructions, but then his footsteps slow down as he realizes he doesn't know how to carry out the instructions and someone else is doing it anyway. In a few days, the other assistants will be using him for work he cannot possibly mess up, like calling the actors from their vanity vans, holding the script pad, or just as a stand-in for a prop or a person. He will have that puzzled look on his face for a few more weeks. He will be bored and maybe text his friends, and the director or a senior AD will spot him exactly at that moment and shout at him for wasting time on the phone. From then on, he will have a serious expression on his face as though he is getting a lot done. A few more days and he will be posting pictures on Facebook. One of him concentrating on the script pad with the director (taken when the director asked him to hold it for a second), one of him with his eye in the camera viewfinder or sitting in front of the monitor (taken when everyone else is on a break). He will be ragged a bit, shouted at and ignored. A couple of movies down the line, he will be doing the same to another young boy or girl.

The experienced ADs are making notes, running behind the director, jotting down edit reports, revising dialogues with the actors. They get shouted at for any glitch, they get compliments when they do it right, they are the strings with which the director holds the set together.

The set assistants are making some last-minute changes. The capable ones can transform a place in a few hours. A kitchen turns into a bedroom; a bedroom turns into an office. The audio guy is in one corner with his small recording device. The boom rod guy is his constant companion. After live sound was introduced, these guys have become indispensable. The audio person needs to give the cue that the audio is rolling once the camera starts to roll and

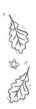

only then can the shoot commence. The cue is usually shouted across because he sits about ten feet away from the camera. The boom rod guy with his long rod and mike needs to hold it in such a way that the dialogues and sounds are captured but the mike and he are never in the frame. I have seen these poor fellows in all sorts of positions to accomplish this feat. Hanging on to pillars, lying on the floor, under tables, behind chairs, clinging to posts or walls, hanging from the roof. I am sure they would not feel out of place in an advanced yoga class. Right now the boom guy is hanging from a half-open door to record the actor speaking right below him. He could fall into the middle of the scene at any moment, but he hangs on with tenacity and I am fascinated by his balancing skills on a swinging door.

Now I come to the most amusing character—the friend. They come along with an artist and stay the entire day doing nothing. Most sit around and chat with anyone who is free. They eat with the artist they have come with, take numerous photos, text or play games on their phone and leave when their friend does. This happens the following day and the day after that too. I cannot imagine why anybody would voluntarily sit around doing nothing. I guess they are company for the actor friend, but I still find this culture of a useless entourage weird.

One junior actor is having trouble with his lines. He just doesn't seem to be able to get it right. Numerous retakes later, everyone is irritated with him. There is no one around who can take his place and hiring a replacement could take days. He is not inexperienced and this shouldn't be happening. The senior actors are all waiting for him to get it right before they can do their part. I can see the man is getting on my husband's nerves, but he is not showing it. I am impressed. He realizes it is a difficult situation that calls for patience and maybe prayers that the guy will get it right soon. He has already pushed the schedule back and it looks like it's going to be one long night.

Before my blood pressure goes through the roof at the actor's clumsiness, I turn away, looking for a quiet spot, and notice a chap working silently. He is in charge of the monitor on which the shot taken by the camera can be seen or played back. His only job is to align the monitor with the camera. He picks it up and positions it near the camera but outside the frame, and plugs it into the electrical board. This happens every time the camera moves. He also plays back whatever has been shot for the director or the actor. He does this without engaging in any conversation.

The guy with the clapboard runs in front of the camera and calls out the take number and I come out of my reverie. My dear husband moves away from the camera. He doesn't stand still for a single moment, not even taking time to sit while the camera is rolling. I have never seen him more focussed or as serious as he is right now. Later that night, he tells me it's a totally different experience for him. As an actor, he isn't responsible for anything other than his acting. Now the whole movie rests on his shoulders. It is a huge responsibility.

I am confident of his abilities. He lives and breathes cinema. I know he has the whole film running scene by scene in his head. There is a clarity and efficiency in the way he shoots the scene, which is beautiful to watch. He knows exactly what he wants from the angles and the characters. He doesn't shoot many extra scenes and there is no confusion or doubt. This is where he differs considerably from me as a director. I am constantly beset with doubts and misgivings. I shoot extra angles and extra scenes that may come in handy during editing or if I discover something wrong later. He already has the edited version in his head. In all honesty, I cannot even compare my style with his. I do not have

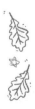

that kind of focus or clarity of thought. I cannot give so much of myself even when I am the director. A parallel reel would be running through my head if things were to go out of schedule or even otherwise—home, kids, kitchen...

There is an earnestness about Dhanush that has not jaded a bit, even after all these years in the industry. When I ask him the secret, he says, 'I have had no life outside cinema. I don't know anything else.' I know he is being honest when he says this. Except when he is with his family, friends, or on the sets of a movie, he is rather ill at ease.

The actor still hasn't got his lines right. Deciding that it's time for me to head back, I look around, but can't will myself to move. Then I realize I don't want to leave. This is where I always want to be, in the midst of this madness called movies.

A Different Role—
Making a Difference

We are all insulated in some way or the other, but some ground realities are hard to ignore, particularly in our country, where the track record when it comes to women is not something to be proud of. I was fairly young when it first occurred to me that I was extremely lucky to have been born to my parents. My father's success afforded us an easy childhood and my sister and I were always treated with respect, unlike many girls of our age. My parents and grandparents never let me feel inferior because I was a girl child. My parents had two daughters and they did not wish for any more children, boys or girls. They have never shown regret in word or deed over not having a boy, and my sister and I were brought up to be independent.

My grandmother was a strong woman who instilled the same in me pretty early in life. One quality that I took away from her was her confidence and sense of achievement. She did not have a career, but what she achieved with her children, with helping others to achieve success, and the many interests she had outside home and family, stayed with me. At the same time, I had inspiring people all around me, who consciously or indirectly drilled into my psyche the importance of financial

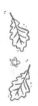

independence. So, when the opportunity arose to make a difference, I grabbed it.

Giving back has been part of my family's way of life ever since I can remember. Appa's numerous acts of charity that he never spoke about and my mother's work with underprivileged children taught us that it was our responsibility to contribute to society, especially since we were so blessed ourselves. There is a much used and abused line from *Spiderman* about power and responsibility. With the little power that I had along with the reflected power from Appa and Dhanush, I decided I wanted to make a difference, however small the impact would turn out to be.

I had been following the work of UN Women for some time, mostly because of the advocacy done by its goodwill ambassadors from India—tennis player Sania Mirza and actor Farhan Akhtar. I admired the way in which the organization was steadily working towards closing the gender gap. I mostly followed them on social media and in a happy turn of events, the same media helped me connect with them. One thing led to another and on a rainy Monday morning, I was honoured to be appointed UN Women's Advocate for Gender Equality and Women's Empowerment in India. Certain things happen without much planning because they are meant to be. This was one of them. And I do not take my role lightly. My husband, my mother, sister and friends were all there to support me at the event. It was they who set the first example in my journey. That of unconditional support.

As I stood there and spoke, I wished a lot more people could hear me, and know about the wonderful work being done by UN Women. After all, that was the point of being an advocate.

So here goes.

Acceptance Speech

I am honoured to stand here before you and accept this prestigious task. Thank you, UN Women, Mrs Lakshmi Puri and Dr Rebecca Tavares for selecting me as the UN Women Goodwill Advocate. I look at the list of UN Women's goodwill ambassadors and I can only think that this honour is fortuitous for me. A reminder I will bear as long as I continue to serve.

As part of this felicitation, I was requested to share my thoughts on the equality of women and what it means to be the UN Women Goodwill Advocate. Bear with me and I promise to keep this short.

As my first reaction, I thought that I should focus on issues pertaining to inequality, the lack of a level playing field, how women struggle every day, how patriarchy (sometimes assisted by other women) keeps a majority of us subjugated. That was making me bitter. That's when I paused to reflect.

I realize we women do a great disservice to ourselves and to all the men who support us by focusing on the grimness of the reality we are faced with. I know it is a hard reality. I know it is unfair where we find ourselves, to say the least. But this is not just about how unfair the world is or how hard our struggles are.

This is also the time to look back and celebrate how far we have come. I am a proud and happy woman. Given a choice, I would want to be born as a woman again. (That is, assuming there is something called rebirth.) That means something. It means I am not angry and bitter. It means my life has thankfully not

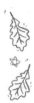

been all that bad. It means that I feel respected by the men and women in my life, and that they respect my aspirations and the choices I make. I am conscious of the fact that I am part of a privileged minority. I am also conscious that there are many women who struggle every day to be accepted. Some, or maybe most, struggle for basic human dignity. But my point is this—more than half a century ago we did not believe that this was possible: a room full of women meeting and discussing how to be masters of our own destiny. A meeting such as this, were it to have been held then, we probably would have been considered revolutionaries or faced resistance. Some may have viewed such a gathering as a gathering of visionaries, maybe. Now, we stand here without any fear of persecution. While we do respect and continue to encourage the men who support us, we are now in a position to speak for ourselves. We have come a long way indeed. Some of us might not see this to be much. But I urge you to celebrate. Small victories and quiet celebrations are very important in a long journey. They teach us not to lose heart, they help us to believe that perseverance and hard work can and do take us far. While we focus on the task ahead, it is also important to cherish what we have achieved until now. Remember, when the cause is just and fair, we will always find people stepping up to lend their support. Sometimes women, and sometimes men.

So, where do we stand? I see that the role and status of women in India have gone through many changes through the millennia. From a position of equal standing in ancient times to a decline in status in medieval times and to a push for equality in the modern era. What strikes me as odd is that while women have held high offices and exalted positions such as the Office of the President of India, Prime Minister, Governor, Chief Minister, Speaker of the Lok Sabha, while we have leading authors, entrepreneurs, CEOs, actresses, directors, etc., yet the resistance to listening to a woman continues. It is odd that despite all that women have achieved, we are required to prove ourselves again and again. Not just have to prove ourselves as capable of doing a job but capable of even being considered for a job. I am yet to make sense of that.

While on that, I do want to mention the environment that we find ourselves in. Rape, acid attacks, forced prostitution, dowry killings and violent victimization. I understand that India is ranked as the worst G-20 country to be born into as a woman and one of the worst countries for women in the world. That is appalling, and it's difficult to understand how we find ourselves here. How can we be one of the worst countries for women to live in and yet have women achievers in many diverse fields? How can women continue to be the backbone of our rural economy and yet not feel at home in our country?

So, what needs to be done? Create awareness? Better opportunities? Inclusive education? Force a revolution? Inculcate self-respect? Probably, we need all of that and something more. If we believe that this organization and each one of us are here to make a difference, let's

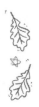

chalk out a plan. Nothing noteworthy, I believe, can be achieved without a plan, focus and an indomitable spirit. Every action we take has to be measurable and result-oriented. And capable of being achieved within a set timeline. I pledge to do my part. Create awareness, support causes identified by the organization with my time and resources. I will do my best to be the woman I want to see and admire in our country. I will do my best to support and encourage women to push themselves, to achieve all that they want to do.

We have covered some distance. Today, we stand by ourselves, believe in ourselves, and are not afraid to voice our views. Those simple acts have taken many years to come true. We often do not see that. Yes, it is a work in progress. Not all of us can claim to be there. For those mothers, sisters and daughters who cannot, we will stand by you. Remember, we can be leaders of men and when we are inspired by a man, we will not hesitate to follow as well.

I take inspiration from each one of you in this room and from the silent struggles of the generations that have gone before us. What we resolve to do now may not bear results today. Or even tomorrow. But we do it nevertheless, in the hope that it will create a better future. Not just for us as women but also for our men.

Let us not fail to look back and count our achievements so we can continue to move forward. Let us not forget that many sacrifices were made so we can be here and that freedom does not come easy. This recognition is a way of saying thank you to everyone who believed in us.

Life is probably art. And in art, the perfect balance is utopian and probably that can never be. But that does not mean we should stop striving to achieve it. Sometimes the balance tilts, sometimes what we ask for and fight for could unfairly prejudice someone. Let us not be indifferent to that. The purpose of any movement is to be an inclusive one.

I leave you with this quote: never think there is anything impossible for the soul. It is the greatest heresy to think so. If there is sin, this is the only sin: to say that you are weak, or others are weak.

Thank you for your patience and for being here with us. Godspeed to us!

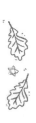

Dance with Me

30 September 2016
6:30 p.m.

The lights are blinding. The hall is packed and the dressing room is bustling with children of all age groups and a few adults. Thick makeup is being lathered on faces and eyes are being beautifully lined with dark kohl. Enthusiastic mothers are handing out temple jewellery from bags hanging from their shoulders. Jewellery that will soon sparkle on their children's arms, foreheads and ears. Fresh jasmine is being braided into hair and red alta is being painted on tiny feet and hands. A mother is supplying coffee and kathi rolls to all the participants. Most of them take just a bite and a sip, unable to eat or drink with just thirty minutes left for the show to start.

It is my dance guru Meenakshi Chittaranjan's silver jubilee celebrations and a hundred dancers are prepping to do their bit on stage. A couple of months earlier, Meena Athai (that is what I have been calling her for years now) had asked me to be part of the celebrations. It was almost seven and a half years since I danced. Both of us knew I was completely out of practice. When Linga turned two, I wanted to get back to dancing, but it didn't happen. I kept procrastinating and would think about it only when I bumped into my guru on various occasions. I would promise to come for class that week and then forget about it. It happened so many times that Meena Athai would smile knowingly every time I said it. She knew I was not going to turn up and had given up on me coming back to dance. So when the call came, I said I would love to be part of it and that I would act as a compère for the show. She did not suggest otherwise and hung up. I was relieved but didn't miss the slight disappointment in her voice. She had wanted me to dance.

I still remember the first time I set foot in her home. It was a sprawling house, untouched by modernity. I remember walking through a long narrow corridor that opened into a large hall. The hall had a big old dining table at one end and a brass Nataraja statue standing tall at the other. The space in between was empty. At the feet of the Nataraja statue was a mat with a stick and a wooden board to beat the rhythm when dancing. I was with my aunt that day. When Amma had told my aunt about my interest in dance, she had suggested we speak to Meenakshi ma'am, who was a friend of hers. My mother wanted me to learn the classical form and my aunt Sudha thought Meena Athai would be the best person to teach me.

She was upstairs when we arrived, and I can still picture the green sari and minimal jewellery that she wore. It was Vijayadashami and she had been meeting students since early in the morning. She looked tired, but her expression was warm and welcoming. She initiated me into her fold and my lifelong affair with dance began.

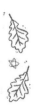

Soon that house became my second home. I couldn't wait to go to dance class. Meena Athai understood my background and the baggage that came with it. She knew exactly when I needed discipline and when I needed some space. As I grew up,

I had started to build pretty strong defences against everyone around me who wasn't family. I was paranoid that they had other agendas when they sought to make friends with me. With my guru, those defences crumbled. I was instantly at ease. I don't call her my teacher or guru, she became my Athai, my aunt. A support system, guide and friend all rolled into one.

Apart from the fondness for my teacher, I also adored her mother, Savitri Paati. She was a big woman, full of life and an energy that would light up everyone around her. Not once did I see her sad or low on enthusiasm for life. A beauty even in her later years, she was dominating and endearing at the same time. She would pull up a chair and sit down to watch us during our classes. She would be there when my guru was practising with her master too, and she took interest in every aspect of her daughter's dance career, encouraging and pushing her to do better. I believe she was the driving force behind my guru's success. Every time I walked into their home, she would greet me with a warm hug. As I started spending more time with her, practicing for the advanced levels, she and I became closer. I could never leave without having a couple of dosas and her specialty—cold coffee. I saw my own grandmother in her and loved her almost as much. The confidence and authority she wielded was comforting, particularly since I had lost my own grandmother.

My guru taught the Pandanalloor style of Bharatanatyam. Pandanalloor is a village close to Tanjavur, where the style originated. Clean lines, intricate footwork, purity of movement and grace are just some of the characteristics of this style. Bharatanatyam has come a long way, with the families that were the original proponents of a particular style taking up steady jobs while dancers like my teacher took on the responsibility of continuing the tradition. Most teachers are inflexible when it comes to training, but Meena Athai understood my compulsions and the flexibility I needed because of my family. The classes would be held early in the morning, or late in the evening, and most often it would be just me and her. She wasn't taking on too many students at the time, but later they demolished the old house and a new dance hall was built, adjacent to the new house, where groups of students could be taught. I continued my classes there until I got married.

The lights are now on me. I look out into the audience. I know all my loved ones including my husband are sitting there, eyes on me. Beside me, my companion dancers including my Meena Athai sparkle brilliantly, ready to start. I had started this journey when I walked into Meena Athai's home and this was just another step, long overdue in my lifelong quest to learn the art of Bharatanatyam.

The music begins and I dance.

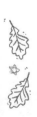

Looking Ahead

There is an English rhyme, 'Tinker Tailor', which lists various occupations. My life has been a bit like that. When I was young I wanted to be a lawyer, later I wanted to be a stay-at-home mother. I learned dance and then I directed movies and now I have donned a new hat, that of a writer. In between all this I've had to play the role of a superstar's daughter and a star's wife.

The lawyer bug was squashed as I grew up, but I couldn't escape the movies. When you grow up in an atmosphere saturated by one thing, then marry into it too, you end up creating plans around it. Like a sponge that absorbs water and remains wet even though you try to squeeze it dry, movies got into my marrow and refused to leave. Growing up seeing movies being made, then watching my husband's unending passion for movie-making, I gravitated towards it. Observing Appa's spirituality and Amma's need to make a difference, I started to want to give back and do more with my life. I came up with excuses along the way, but at each turn, there were counters to those excuses staring right into my eyes and egging me on.

Appa did not want us to be in the movie business. He had seen its dark side. He worried that we might want to become actors. Little did he know that my sister and I didn't want to be among the ship's crew, we wanted to captain it.

As the child of a living legend, people would often ask, 'Why do you even try? You can put your feet up, enjoy the life your father has built for you and the comfort your husband provides, and let things come to you. Take care of the home, shop, bring up your kids and enjoy life.'

I wish!

Most people don't understand that being a homemaker is a full-time vocation in itself. I chose to be a homemaker and then do a little extra. My dreams of becoming a lawyer, dancer, mother, film-maker, author and an advocate for women's rights have all come to fruition in one way or another. I have been blessed but I need to keep moving.

They say god gives challenges only to those who can handle them. A hassle-free day-to-day life, a fully functioning home and happy children are achievements in themselves. But most women, either to challenge themselves or due to external challenges, have to do more. I have my own battles to fight, from trying to resist my appetite for sweets to trying to make my own mark in the world. And I must confess, temptation when it comes to food is the hardest to overcome!

I would like to do more for the cause of women and I have got the perfect platform with my role as a UN Women's advocate. I would also like to do more for the industry that has nurtured me from birth. We are currently working on a three-part series on the unsung heroes of the industry. The first part deals with stunt men and women. Very rarely do our movies not feature stunts, yet the people who make them possible are ignored. They put their lives on the line, yet there is no recognition, no insurance coverage and very little compensation. The project started with a documentary, and went on with a petition to add stunt choreography as a category for the National awards. It is a surprising omission that must change.

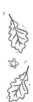

The second part of the series deals with junior artistes. They enter the field with stars in their eyes, but are soon struggling for survival and it is only their passion for cinema that keeps them going. The third and last part will delve into the lives of background dancers. Song and dance have been such a staple of our movies, but these dancers are often the most underpaid in the industry. This trilogy is a tribute to these people who are not acknowledged, but are such an integral part of movie-making.

These are my plans. I hope I can look back and say things worked out right and I did the right thing by all those I set out to do it for, and with.

For the rest, there's god and family.

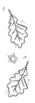

Acknowledgements

To the men.

My grandfather, who pushed me to be passionate about language. Those lovely evenings he spent reading to me, the early morning newspaper headlines we discussed together, the lovely letters he sent later in life, they laid the foundation for this book.

Appa, words cannot do justice to the bond we share. Thank you for the great genes!

Dhanush, my friend and companion for life, whose encouragement made me truly spread my wings.

My two beautiful sons, who have taught me the true meaning of life. I hope constantly that I am worthy of their love and that they grow up to be strong men who respect the women in their lives.

My grandmother, for making me believe that I can achieve, my mother and sister for their love, and my friends for being my eternal support system.

This book couldn't have happened without the people I am going to mention next. Aditi Ravindranath, for having faith in me and recognizing that there was a writer in me. Amritha Dinesh, for helping me put it together and move ahead, keeping the deadlines in mind. Mr Baradwaj Rangan, who instantly put me on to the right people. Karthika V.K. at HarperCollins India, who was extremely encouraging and helpful. I thank you all from the warmest part of my heart.